Praise for *Johns Hopkins Evidence-Based Practice for Nurses and Healthcare Professionals,* Fourth Edition

"The fourth edition is an exceptional guide to ensure evidence-based practice is a core competency of nurses. The authors effectively communicate actionable strategies for clinicians to determine which EBP projects will yield measurable practice improvements. They artfully address the cultural and behavioral needs and motivations that influence the success of teams and organizations as they implement EBP changes. Through the use of well-defined tools, users will accurately evaluate evidence, develop strong implementation plans, and understand pathways for dissemination."

–Jennifer Williams, PhD, RN, ACNS-BC, CEN, CCRN-K
Director of Nursing Practice, Research and Professional Development
The University of Kansas Health System

"*Johns Hopkins Evidenced-Based Practice for Nurses and Healthcare Professionals* is an excellent resource that can be utilized to create an EBP culture. The authors present the EBP process in ways that staff can understand so it is not overwhelming. As the facilitator for our EBP & Research Council, we chose the Johns Hopkins EBP model, and it was the best decision we made!"

–Elena Vidrine, MSN, RN, NEA-BC, RN-BC
Director of Nursing Professional Development
Children's Hospital New Orleans

"As the nurse anesthesiology (NA) profession continues to fully transition all NA educational programs (NAEP) to entry-level doctoral degrees, the crucial question is: How do we achieve the scholarship requirement? There are challenges and barriers in the completion of the academic piece, with an additional question of: How do we marry evidence and clinical practice? As an NAEP practice doctorate, we, as clinical practitioners, academicians, and researchers, do not want to overstretch our already overwhelmed healthcare systems. Rather, our primary goal is to improve clinical outcomes and keep our patients safe. *Johns Hopkins Evidence-Based Practice for Nurses and Healthcare Professionals,* Fourth Edition, systematically and thoroughly describes the PET process: how to identify the practice question, examine the most recent evidence, and guide the practitioner to efficiently translate the evidence as applicable to clinical practice. The problem, intervention, comparison, and outcome (PICO) model methodically guides all researchers from all levels of expertise using this comprehensive evidence-based process. The Johns Hopkins EBP model is the best fit for our NAEP since it not only streamlines the academic scholarship piece but also connects what is germane to day-to-day clinical practice: to promote patient safety."

–Jose D. Castillo III, PhD, MSNA, CRNA, APRN
t Professor of Nurse Anesthesia
Texas Wesleyan University

"Another great update. I have used this book for 10 years as a text in a nursing course. The additions and upgrades including search content, databases, and use of forms are important revisions. The inclusion of interprofessional focus aligns with current healthcare needs for evidence-based practice. Practicing nurses find the Johns Hopkins Model easy to use to enable improving care. The book can be used in a variety of healthcare programs and different degrees."

–Martha Jenner, MSN, RNC-OB
Professor, RN-to-BSN Program
Florida SouthWestern State College

"My organization's rehab department received education on the Johns Hopkins Model a few years ago from our Director of Evidence-Based Practice and Nursing Research. Since that time, we have included the tool as part of our rehab department's evidence-based practice education. The book's appendices provide a step-by-step approach for using the model for large- or small-scale EBP initiatives, such as Appendices E and F for identifying evidence level and quality for journal club discussions. Rehab staff within my organization have used the tool for appraising and summarizing literature to answer clinical questions or contribute to standards of care. The tool has been used to address therapy-specific clinical questions but also in collaboration with nursing staff for interdisciplinary care inquiries. One example that comes to mind is a project between speech therapy and nursing staff to identify risk factors for dysphagia after cervical surgery. It is valuable to have a model that can be used across the interdisciplinary team to approach EBP with a consistent process for addressing clinical questions. I am encouraged to see the authors call out and support the importance of interdisciplinary collaboration for the EBP process in the newest edition of this book."

–Ashley J. Peters, PT, DPT
Board-Certified Neurologic Clinical Specialist
WellSpan Health

"This fourth edition of this foundational book provides yet more helpful and valuable advances in clarifying and applying a complex concept to empower our healthcare teams in effectively utilizing evidence-based practice. Grateful to see the model and tools continue to evolve based on user feedback—the book feels as essential, practical, and helpful as ever!"

–Jen Bonamer, PhD, RN, NPD-BC, AHN-BC (Pronouns: She/Her)
Clinical Nurse Researcher
Nursing Prof'l Development – Research Specialist
Education, Prof'l Development & Research Dept.
Sarasota Memorial Health Care System

Praise for *Johns Hopkins Nursing Evidence-Based Practice: Model and Guidelines,* Third Edition

"Part of the challenge of teaching the EBP process is how to keep it simple so frontline staff can understand the process and stop seeing it as so complex that only nurses pursuing graduate studies can comprehend. That is where this book comes in handy. The Johns Hopkins Nursing Evidence-Based Practice PET (Practice question, Evidence, and Translation) process is explained in an understandable, guiding manner from beginning to end. In addition to helping one be organized, the tools are an integral part of further understanding the EBP components. The exemplars make EBP 'doable' and thus relatable. It is impressive that cited EBP projects were implemented by a single nurse or team of nurses, ranging from frontline staff to multidisciplinary teams, and including partnering physicians. The book also covers how to overcome barriers to EBP and how to sustain change achieved from implementing the process. This book gives nurses the knowledge and power to disseminate EBP, and it is not far-fetched to expect EBP to be a nursing habit."

–Ruth Bala-Kerr, MSN, RN, CNS, CPHQ, NE-BC
Director, Clinical Professional Development, Harbor-UCLA Medical Center

"As a clinical nurse leader and EBP champion, I absolutely love the *Johns Hopkins Nursing Evidence-Based Practice: Model and Guidelines* book; it is my all-time favorite resource book on the subject. I had the opportunity to attend a Johns Hopkins EBP boot camp, and while reading this book, I felt as though I was having that amazing experience again! This book is easy to read and a great tool for nurses on any level of proficiency. I recommend it as a practical way to integrate EBP into any practice environment."

–Kimberly M. Barnes, MSN, RN, CNL
Clinical Nurse Leader, Patient Care Services

"In 2006, our organization chose to adopt the Johns Hopkins Nursing Evidence-Based Practice Model because of its ease of use and its tools for nurses with diverse educational backgrounds. With each new edition, the authors improve the quality and function of this model. This third edition provides further depth and clarification with the addition of a new chapter, 'Lessons From Practice: Using the JHNEBP Tools,' and translation tools that provide clear, concise instruction. We will continue to use this book as a resource for our nurses and allied health professionals in developing their knowledge and skills in identification and translation of evidence into daily clinical and administrative decision-making."

–Barbara L. Buchko, DNP, RNC-MNN
Director of Evidence-Based Practice and Nursing Research,
WellSpan Health

"In early 2000, The Johns Hopkins Hospital (JHH) Post Anesthesia Care Unit (PACU) was very fortunate to be the pilot site for the Johns Hopkins Nursing Evidence-Based Practice Model. PACU nurses from inpatient and ambulatory settings were invited to participate. There was a sense of staff reluctance and lack of appreciation for what their involvement meant. Seeing the nurses' active engagement in the pilot and outcome was every nurse manager's dream. Using evidence in making decisions became a reality. *Johns Hopkins Nursing Evidence-Based Practice: Model and Guidelines,* Third Edition, captures the essence of nursing excellence in practice. This book illustrates the barriers in today's nursing practice in developing critical thinking and competence; it provides the structure, process, tools, and measurement of outcomes for proficiency levels ranging from nursing students to leaders and for every setting. I am most grateful to Johns Hopkins for its nursing leadership in the culture of inquiry."

–Dina A. Krenzischek, PhD, RN, CPAN, CFRE, FAAN
Director of Professional Practice, Mercy Medical Center

"*Johns Hopkins Nursing Evidence-Based Practice: Model and Guidelines* is very practical, with clarity about how to determine evidence levels and additional factors that influence practice. The new model is active and interrelating. Support materials available to end users are reasonably priced, practical, and helpful to bedside nurses who conduct evidence-based practice projects. We use these materials for EBP improvement, EBP internships, and nurse residency. Model elements are easy to understand and explain. The detailed, stepwise progression from forming a team and clinical question to disseminating findings guides a comprehensive and systematic approach to EBP. The focus on translation of best evidence into practice addresses one of the most challenging and critical phases of EBP. Our Organizational Nursing Research Council adopted the JHNEBP Model and has been using the support materials for almost 10 years. The exemplars are helpful in supporting learning. Our hospital purchased the ebook, and we look forward to updating to the third edition."

–Debra Haas Stavarski, PhD, MS, RN
Director of Nursing Research, Reading Hospital, Reading Health System

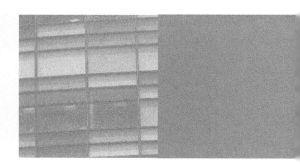

Johns Hopkins
Evidence-Based Practice for Nurses and Healthcare Professionals
Fourth Edition

Model and Guidelines

Deborah Dang, PhD, RN, NEA-BC
Sandra L. Dearholt, DNP, RN, NEA-BC
Kim Bissett, PhD, MBA, RN
Judy Ascenzi, DNP, RN, CCRN-K
Madeleine Whalen, MSN/MPH, RN, CEN

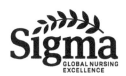
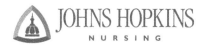

Copyright © 2022 by Sigma Theta Tau International Honor Society of Nursing

All rights reserved. This book is protected by copyright. No part of it may be reproduced, stored in a retrieval system, or transmitted in any form or by any means, electronic, mechanical, photocopying, recording, or otherwise, without written permission from the publisher. Any trademarks, service marks, design rights, or similar rights that are mentioned, used, or cited in this book are the property of their respective owners. Their use here does not imply that you may use them for a similar or any other purpose.

This book is not intended to be a substitute for the medical advice of a licensed medical professional. The author and publisher have made every effort to ensure the accuracy of the information contained within at the time of its publication and shall have no liability or responsibility to any person or entity regarding any loss or damage incurred, or alleged to have incurred, directly or indirectly, by the information contained in this book. The author and publisher make no warranties, express or implied, with respect to its content, and no warranties may be created or extended by sales representatives or written sales materials. The author and publisher have no responsibility for the consistency or accuracy of URLs and content of third-party websites referenced in this book.

Sigma Theta Tau International Honor Society of Nursing (Sigma) is a nonprofit organization whose mission is developing nurse leaders anywhere to improve healthcare everywhere. Founded in 1922, Sigma has more than 135,000 active members in over 100 countries and territories. Members include practicing nurses, instructors, researchers, policymakers, entrepreneurs, and others. Sigma's more than 540 chapters are located at more than 700 institutions of higher education throughout Armenia, Australia, Botswana, Brazil, Canada, Colombia, Croatia, England, Eswatini, Ghana, Hong Kong, Ireland, Israel, Italy, Jamaica, Japan, Jordan, Kenya, Lebanon, Malawi, Mexico, the Netherlands, Nigeria, Pakistan, Philippines, Portugal, Puerto Rico, Scotland, Singapore, South Africa, South Korea, Sweden, Taiwan, Tanzania, Thailand, the United States, and Wales. Learn more at www.sigmanursing.org.

Sigma Theta Tau International
550 West North Street
Indianapolis, IN, USA 46202

To request a review copy for course adoption, order additional books, buy in bulk, or purchase for corporate use, contact Sigma Marketplace at 888.654.4968 (US/Canada toll-free), +1.317.687.2256 (International), or solutions@sigmamarketplace.org.

To request author information, or for speaker or other media requests, contact Sigma Marketing at 888.634.7575 (US/Canada toll-free) or +1.317.634.8171 (International).

ISBN: 9781948057875
EPUB ISBN: 9781948057882
PDF ISBN: 9781948057899
MOBI ISBN: 9781948057905

Library of Congress Control Number: 2021938845

Third Printing, 2024

Publisher: Dustin Sullivan
Acquisitions Editor: Emily Hatch
Project Editor: Rebecca Senninger
Copy Editor: Erin Geile
Cover Designer: Rebecca Batchelor
Interior Design/Page Layout: Rebecca Batchelor

Managing Editor: Carla Hall
Publications Specialist: Todd Lothery
Development Editor: Rebecca Senninger
Proofreader: Gill Editorial Services
Indexer: Larry Sweazy

DEDICATION

This book is dedicated to nurses and healthcare professionals everywhere in whatever setting they practice—who are committed to excellence in patient care based on best available evidence.

ACKNOWLEDGMENTS

We would like to acknowledge the insight and expertise of the authors of the first edition (2007) of *Johns Hopkins Nursing Evidence-Based Practice: Model and Guidelines*: Robin P. Newhouse, PhD, RN, NE-BC, FAAN; Sandra L. Dearholt, DNP, RN, NEA-BC; Stephanie S. Poe, DNP, RN; Linda C. Pugh, PhD, RNC, CNE, FAAN; and Kathleen M. White, PhD, RN, NEA-BC, FAAN.

The foundational work of these experts transformed evidence-based practice into a process that promotes autonomy and provides frontline nurses with the competencies and tools to apply the best evidence to improve patient care. The profession as a whole is indebted to them.

About the Authors

Deborah Dang, PhD, RN, NEA-BC

Deborah Dang is the Senior Director of Nursing Inquiry and Research at the Johns Hopkins Health System. She developed the strategic vision for evidence-based practice (EBP) for Johns Hopkins Nursing and built an infrastructure that has enabled the transformation to practice based on evidence. In her role as Director of Nursing for Practice, Education, Research at The Johns Hopkins Hospital, she led and championed nursing professional practice, cultivating its growth from the initial model development to final implementation. She cocreated, with clinical nurses and nurse leaders, The Johns Hopkins Hospital Professional Practice Model: clinical advancement program, professional development for frontline leaders and staff, salaried compensation, shared governance, and evidence-based practice, thus building an infrastructure to continually advance nursing excellence. As a health services researcher, her funded studies focused on disruptive behavior, positive psychology, and mindful leadership. She received the inaugural New Investigator Award for the AcademyHealth Interdisciplinary Research Group on Nursing Issues, is a Fellow of the Wharton Nurse Executive Program, and was recognized as a Distinguished EBP Trailblazer by Fuld National Institute for EBP in 2019. Dang has published, consulted, and presented nationally and internationally on the subject of EBP. She also holds a Joint Appointment with the Johns Hopkins University School of Nursing.

Sandra L. Dearholt, DNP, RN, NEA-BC

Sandra L. Dearholt is Assistant Director of Nursing for the Departments of Neurosciences and Psychiatry Nursing at The Johns Hopkins Hospital. Dearholt has written numerous articles on EBP and has extensive experience in the development and delivery of EBP educational programs. Her areas of interest focus on strategies for incorporating EBP into practice at the bedside, the development of professional practice standards, promoting healthcare staff well-being, and fostering service excellence. She is a coauthor of the first edition of *Johns Hopkins Nursing Evidence-Based Practice: Model and Guidelines* and a contributing author to *Johns Hopkins Nursing Evidence-Based Practice: Implementation and Translation*.

Kim Bissett, PhD, MBA, RN

Kim Bissett is a nurse educator and director of EBP at the Institute for Johns Hopkins Nursing. She was the inaugural Evidence-Based Practice Coordinator at The Johns Hopkins Hospital, following two years of serving as the EBP Fellow. She assisted with the development and publication of the second and third editions of *Johns Hopkins Nursing Evidence-Based Practice: Model and Guidelines*. Bissett has presented and consulted on the topic of evidence-based nursing practice both nationally and internationally. Her research interests include building EBP competencies, self-compassion, and fostering nurse well-being.

Judy Ascenzi, DNP, RN, CCRN-K

Judy Ascenzi is the Director of Pediatric Nursing Programs for Education, Informatics, and Research at the Johns Hopkins Children's Center. She also teaches part time in the Johns Hopkins University School of Nursing's Doctorate of Nursing Practice Program. Ascenzi has presented and consulted nationally on the topic of evidence-based practice. She has served as expert facilitator on many evidence-based practice projects in her pediatric practice setting as well as with her adult colleagues at The Johns Hopkins Hospital. She acts as a project advisor and organizational mentor for many doctoral students utilizing the JHEBP Model as the foundational model for their projects.

Madeleine Whalen, MSN/MPH, RN, CEN

Madeleine Whalen is the Evidence-Based Practice Program Coordinator for the Johns Hopkins Health System. In this role, she supports frontline nursing in completing robust and actionable EBP projects. She began her nursing career in the emergency department while earning her master's degrees in nursing and public health. She continues to work clinically part time and serves as a Clinical Instructor at The Johns Hopkins School of Nursing. Her professional interests include global health, infectious disease, and empowering nurses to advance the profession and science of nursing through inquiry.

About the Contributing Authors

Chapter 1: Evidence-Based Practice: Context, Concerns, and Challenges

Kim Bissett, PhD, MBA, RN

> See Kim Bissett's bio earlier.

Special acknowledgment to previous author Linda C. Pugh, PhD, RN, RNC, FAAN.

Chapter 2: Creating a Supportive EBP Environment

Kathleen White, PhD, RN, NEA-BC, FAAN

> Kathleen White is a Professor at the Johns Hopkins University School of Nursing. White has authored multiple publications on the Johns Hopkins Nursing EBP Model and also consults and presents on this subject. White coauthored the first edition of *Johns Hopkins Nursing Evidence-Based Practice: Model and Guidelines* and coedited *Johns Hopkins Nursing Evidence-Based Practice: Implementation and Translation*.

Deborah Dang, PhD, RN, NEA-BC

> See Deborah Dang's bio earlier.

Chapter 3: The Johns Hopkins Evidence-Based Practice (JHEBP) Model for Nurses and Healthcare Professionals (HCPs) Process Overview

Sandra L. Dearholt, DNP, RN, NEA-BC

> See Sandra L. Dearholt's bio earlier.

Chapter 4: The Practice Question Phase

Judy Ascenzi, DNP, RN, CCRN-K

> See Judy Ascenzi's bio earlier.

Kim Bissett, PhD, MBA, RN

> See Kim Bissett's bio earlier.

Special acknowledgment to previous author Robin P. Newhouse, PhD, RN, NEA-BC, FAAN.

Chapter 5: Searching for Evidence

Rachael Lebo, MLS, AHIP

> Rachael Lebo is an informationist at the Welch Medical Library, Johns Hopkins Medical Institutions. She provides service for the information needs of The Johns Hopkins Hospital, School of Medicine, Bloomberg School of Public Health, and Kennedy Krieger Institute. Lebo has helped nurses with their evidence-based practice and quality improvement research projects in collaboration with the Institute for Johns Hopkins Nursing and Johns Hopkins Hospital Nursing Administration. Lebo also holds an adjunct position at the University Libraries, University of South Dakota. She provides assistance in knowledge translation, evidence-based practice, and quality improvement research projects in collaboration with clinical nurses, faculty, staff, and students at the Sanford School of Medicine and partner institutions.

Carrie Price, MLS

> Carrie Price is the Health Professions Librarian at the Albert S. Cook Library, Towson University. She was previously a clinical informationist at the Welch Medical Library, Johns Hopkins Medical Institutions, where she provided reference and instruction to faculty, students, and staff. She has collaborated with the Institute for Johns Hopkins Nursing and Johns Hopkins Hospital Nursing Administration to help nurses succeed in evidence-based practice, knowledge translation, and quality improvement research projects. Price has a strong interest in user-centered and instructional design.

Stella Seal, MLS

> Stella Seal is the Lead Informationist for the School of Nursing, Hospitals & Health System Services at the Welch Medical Library, Johns Hopkins

Medical Institutions. She has more than 20 years of experience providing information services to the faculty, students, and staff of the Johns Hopkins School of Nursing. Seal has presented numerous instructional sessions on all aspects of database searching and research tools, in addition to her collaborations on grant proposals and systematic reviews.

Madeleine Whalen, MSN/MPH, RN, CEN

See Madeleine Whalen's bio earlier.

Special acknowledgment to previous authors Christina L. Wissinger, PhD, and Elizabeth Scala, MSN, MBA, RN.

Chapter 6: Evidence Appraisal: Research

Madeleine Whalen, MSN/MPH, RN, CEN

See Madeleine Whalen's bio earlier.

Deborah Dang, PhD, RN, NEA-BC

See Deborah Dang's bio earlier.

Special acknowledgment to previous authors Linda Costa, PhD, RN, NEA-BC, and Jennifer Day, PhD, RN.

Chapter 7: Evidence Appraisal: Nonresearch

Michelle Patch, PhD, MSN, APRN-CNS, ACNS-BC

Michelle Patch is an Adult Health Clinical Nurse Specialist and Assistant Professor at the Johns Hopkins School of Nursing. She also maintains an active practice with Johns Hopkins Medicine's Armstrong Institute for Patient Safety and Quality and The Johns Hopkins Hospital's Department of Patient Safety. Patch has held progressive clinical, operational, and safety leadership positions in various inpatient, outpatient, emergency, and austere settings. In these capacities, she has successfully led and coached multiple healthcare teams in evidence-based practice projects. Her scholarly interests include intimate partner violence, assault mechanisms, and workplace violence in healthcare, and she lectures internationally on patient and staff safety-related topics.

Jennifer K. Peterson, PhD, APRN-CNS, CCNS, FAHA

> Jennifer Peterson is a Clinical Nurse Specialist and an Assistant Professor at the Johns Hopkins School of Nursing. Her clinical experience includes the care of infants, children, and adolescents with heart disease and their families in a variety of roles across the spectrum of care settings. As a CNS, she is committed to evidence-based practice and patient safety/quality. Her research interests include developmentally supportive care, long-term outcomes of heart disease in children, and healthcare disparities. She teaches in the prelicensure pediatrics course and in the DNP Clinical Nurse Specialist program.

Nicole L. Mollenkopf, PharmD, MBA, BCPS, BCPPS

> Nicole Mollenkopf is an Assistant Professor and Director of Interprofessional Education at the Johns Hopkins School of Nursing and Patient Safety Specialist at the Armstrong Institute for Patient Safety and Quality. She has served as an expert medication safety consultant both nationally and internationally. Her scholarship focuses on methods to improve the quality and safety of the medication-use process. At the prelicensure and advanced practice nursing levels, she teaches pharmacology with a focus on application of evidence-based principles to improve medication outcomes.

Special acknowledgment to previous authors Hayley D. Mark, PhD, MPH, RN, FAAN, and Hyunjeong Park, PhD, MPH, MSN, RN.

Chapter 8: Translation

Robin P. Newhouse, PhD, RN, NEA-BC, FAAN

> Robin P. Newhouse is Dean of the Indiana University School of Nursing and Indiana University Distinguished Professor. Her research focuses on health system interventions to improve care processes and patient outcomes. She has published extensively on health services improvement interventions, acute care quality issues, and evidence-based practice. Newhouse coauthored the first edition of *Johns Hopkins Nursing Evidence-Based Practice: Model and Guidelines*. She is an elected member of the National Academy of Medicine

and appointed Cochair of the Methodology Committee of the Patient Centered Outcomes Research Institute. She was inducted into the Sigma Theta Tau International Honor Society of Nursing Nurse Researcher Hall of Fame in 2014, received the American Nurses Credentialing Center President's Award in 2015, and was recognized as a Distinguished EBP Trailblazer by Fuld National Institute for EBP in 2019.

Kathleen White, PhD, RN, NEA-BC, FAAN

See Kathleen White's bio earlier.

Chapter 9: Dissemination

Madeleine Whalen, MSN, MPH, RN, CEN

See Madeleine Whalen's bio earlier.

Judy Ascenzi, DNP, RN, CCRN-K

See Judy Ascenzi's bio earlier.

Chapter 10: Exemplars

Kim Bissett, PhD, MBA, RN

See Kim Bissett's bio earlier.

Chapter 11: Lessons From Practice: Using the JHEBP Tools

Kim Bissett, PhD, MBA, RN

See Kim Bissett's bio earlier.

Table of Contents

About the Authors viii
About the Contributing Authors xi
Foreword xxi
Introduction xxiii

Part I Evidence-Based Practice Background 1

1 Evidence-Based Practice: Context, Concerns, and Challenges 3
EBP: Definition 5
The History 6
The Push for EBP 7
EBP and Outcomes 8
EBP and Accountability 8
The Healthcare Clinician's Role in EBP 9
Summary 10
References 10

2 Creating a Supportive EBP Environment 13
Choosing an EBP Model 15
Creating and Facilitating a Supportive EBP Environment 16
Ensuring Committed Organizational Leadership 17
Establishing the Organizational Culture 19
Building Capacity 29
Sustaining the Change 33
Communication Plan 35
Summary 37
References 37

Part II The Johns Hopkins Evidence-Based Practice Model and Guidelines 41

3 The Johns Hopkins Evidence-Based Practice (JHEBP) Model for Nurses and Healthcare Professionals (HCPs) Process Overview 43

The Johns Hopkins Evidence-Based Practice (JHEBP) Model for Nurses and HCPs—Essential Components: Inquiry, Practice, and Learning 44
The JHEBP Model—Description 49
JHEBP PET Process: Practice Question, Evidence, and Translation 54
Summary 66
References 66

Part III Practice Question, Evidence, Translation (PET) 71

4 The Practice Question Phase 73

The Interprofessional EBP Team 74
Clarifying and Describing the Practice Problem 80
Developing and Refining the EBP Question 86
Choosing a Background or Foreground Question 86
Determining the Need for an EBP Project 90
Identifying Stakeholders 95
Summary 96
References 96

5 Searching for Evidence 99

Key Information Formats 100
The Answerable Question 101
EBP Search Examples 102
Selecting Information and Evidence Resources 104
Selecting Resources Outside of the Nursing Literature 106
Creating Search Strategies and Utilizing Free Resources 107
Additional Search Techniques 114
Screening, Evaluating, Revising, and Storing Search Results 115
Summary 118
References 119

Evidence Section...121
  Introduction..121
  Evidence Summary..124
  Evidence Synthesis 124
  Summary..126
  References 127

6 Evidence Appraisal: Research...........................129
  Types of Scientific Research 130
  Types of Research Designs 131
  Systemic Reviews Summaries of Multiple Research
  Studies 141
  Determining the Level of Research Evidence 146
  Appraising the Quality of Research Evidence 147
  Recommendations for Interprofessional Leaders 160
  Summary..160
  References 161

7 Evidence Appraisal: Nonresearch 163
  Summaries of Research Evidence 164
  Organizational Experience...173
  Best Practices Companies 182
  Recommendations for Healthcare Leaders.........................182
  Summary..183
  References 183

8 Translation...189
  Translation Models..190
  Components of the Translation Phase................................196
  Final Steps of the Translation Phase.........................203
  Summary..203
  References 204

9 Dissemination 207
  How to Create a Dissemination Plan..................................208
  Internal Dissemination 209
  External Dissemination...211
  Summary..217
  References 218

Part IV Exemplars 221

10 Exemplars 223

Learning While Going Through the Process of an Evidence-Based Practice Project..223
Prevention of LVAD Driveline Infections 226
Outpatient Palliative Care to Improve Quality of Life and Reduce Symptom Burden and 30-Day Readmissions in Patients With Heart Failure 229
Implementation of a Saline and Pulsatile Flush Procedure for Central Venous Catheters...231
Pressure Injury Prevention in the Surgical ICU 234
Gamification in Nursing Education 237
An Evidence-Based Approach to Creating an EBP Culture 241

Part V Using the JHEBP Tools 245

11 Lessons From Practice: Using the JHEBP Tools ...247

Practice Question and Project Planning..............................247
Evidence 254
Translation..271

Part VI Appendices 277

A PET Process Guide 279
B Question Development Tool 283
C Stakeholder Analysis and Communication Tool 289
D Hierarchy of Evidence Guide................................295
E Research Evidence Appraisal Tool 297
F Nonresearch Evidence Appraisal Tool 307
G Individual Evidence Summary Tool 315
H Synthesis and Recommendations Tool 319
I Translation and Action Planning Tool 325
J Publication Guide..333

Index 337

Foreword

It is with great pride that we introduce the fourth edition of the highly valued Johns Hopkins resource, *Johns Hopkins Evidence-Based Practice for Nurses and Healthcare Professionals: Model & Guidelines.*

While I write this, we are amidst a global health pandemic that has brought into sharp focus the strengths and weaknesses of healthcare systems. Without a doubt, the public and leaders worldwide unequivocally recognize the complexity of patient care. Nurses and other members of healthcare teams are more—now than ever—the advocates for and providers of high-quality, compassionate care.

We have all recently experienced the anxiety related to lack of evidence surrounding COVID-19. This dearth of information has put into stark relief how much we rely on evidence to guide our patient care and make ourselves, our families, and our patients feel safe. The visceral feeling of "not knowing" has highlighted the importance of not only producing high-quality evidence but also rapidly and reliably evaluating and implementing it. Never has evidence-based practice felt more important than now, when we know what it's like not to have it.

Feedback from a wide variety of end users, both clinical and academic, inform the continued development and improvement of the Johns Hopkins EBP Model. While the third edition emphasized the importance of inquiry as the foundation of continuous learning, the fourth edition draws attention to the value-added contributions of EBP as an interprofessional activity to enhance team collaboration and care coordination. EBP initiatives have become more collaborative in nature, and interprofessional teams have been shown to enhance quality outcomes through the integration of varied perspectives, lower costs, and safer patient care. As with previous editions, our goal remains constant and is ever more critical—to build capacity among frontline users to discern best practices from common practices and instill them into the everyday care we provide our patients. This is not just a skill set but a mindset, and it will serve nurses and healthcare team members called upon to create and implement healthcare and public health policies in the years to come.

Once again, I am honored to endorse this continued commitment to evidence-based practice and inquiry that supports healthcare quality, innovation, and nursing leadership around the world.

–Deborah Baker, DNP, ACNP, NEA-BC
Senior Vice President for Nursing, Johns Hopkins Health System
Vice President of Nursing and Patient Care Services,
The Johns Hopkins Hospital

Introduction

The dynamic and competitive US healthcare environment requires healthcare professionals who are accountable to provide efficient and effective care. New evidence is continually surfacing in nursing and medical environments. Consumer pressure and increased patient expectations place an even greater emphasis on the need for healthcare professionals to deliver true evidence-based care in their daily practice.

Johns Hopkins Nursing is steadfastly dedicated to making it easy for frontline nurses, health professionals, and students to use best evidence in their everyday practice. With each edition, we revise based on the honest, frank, and generous feedback we receive from frontline users of the Johns Hopkins Evidence-Based Practice Model from across the globe. We are grateful to those healthcare professionals who have taken the time to provide feedback to improve the clarity and usability of the model in a variety of clinical and academic settings. In this fourth edition, we are excited to be able to share these changes.

The 2021 revised JHEBP Model underscores the need for organizations to cultivate both a spirit of inquiry and an environment of learning that encourages questioning and seeking best evidence and its implementation and adoption in practice. Although our model was developed, tested, and implemented by and for nurses, we have had numerous requests and feedback from other health professionals to use the Hopkins model. Thus, we introduce the fourth edition with a new title—*Johns Hopkins Evidence-Based Practice for Nurses and Healthcare Professionals*. This change reflects the growing evidence base of the importance for interprofessional collaboration and teamwork, particularly when addressing complex care issues such as those often tackled by EBP teams.

In this edition, our overarching aim is to provide practical and pragmatic explanations, approaches, and tools to guide and support teams engaging in EBP projects:

- We explicitly reflected the interprofessional nature of the EBP process and its use by all disciplines who serve, interact with, and care for those who seek services.
- We revised the flow of the book chapters across the sections to reflect the progression of steps in the EBP process.
- We included a new introduction for the evidence section that includes a background on use of evidence hierarchies, tips for differentiating research from quality improvement, and further explanation of the summary and synthesis steps in the evidence process.
- We made significant enhancements to the appendices by including flowcharts, decision supports, and greater specificity in the directions.
- We provided real-world examples for how to complete all tools using feedback from our global users as well as tried and tested helpful hints.
- We added a new chapter to expand and amplify strategies for dissemination that includes how to create a dissemination plan, audience-specific recommendations for internal and external dissemination venues, details of the pros and cons of different types of dissemination, guidance on submitting manuscripts for publication, and an overview of the journal review process.
- Chapter-specific enhancements:
    - Chapter 3: Defines critical thinking and clinical reasoning and differentiates their use in the PET process
    - Chapter 4: Outlines stakeholder selection criteria and an algorithm to determine the need for an EBP project
    - Chapter 5: Includes new information on the literature screening process to navigate a large number of results

- Chapter 6: Provides useful clarifications of research approaches, designs, and methods with a focus on frontline staff as the target audience
- Chapter 8: Includes revised synthesis and translation steps; assesses risk prior to translation; prioritizes translation models accessible to frontline staff with a focus on the QI methodology and PDSA; and describes an expanded list of outcome measures to determine the success of an EPB project

The fourth edition honors the imperative first established by M. Adelaide Nutting, Assistant Superintendent of Nurses at The Johns Hopkins Hospital, Principal of the Johns Hopkins School of Nursing, and pioneer in the development of nursing education:

"We need to realize and affirm a view that 'medicine' is one of the most difficult of arts. Compassion may provide the motive, but knowledge is our only working power ... surely we will not be satisfied with merely perpetuating methods and traditions; surely we should be more and more involved with creating them."

Evidence-Based Practice Background

1 Evidence-Based Practice: Context, Concerns, and Challenges 3

2 Creating a Supportive EBP Environment. 13

Evidence-Based Practice: Context, Concerns, and Challenges

To meet the needs of the modern healthcare system, the Institute of Medicine (IOM), now the National Academy of Medicine, published a set of five core competencies required of each health professional. This is not an exhaustive list but represents those competencies common among a variety of health professionals and those most important to advancing healthcare. These competencies included providing patient-centered care, working in interdisciplinary teams, applying quality improvement, utilizing informatics, and employing evidence-based practice (IOM, 2003). As a core competency, evidence-based practice (EBP) represents a significant skill for nurses and other healthcare providers who have considerable influence on healthcare decisions and improving the quality and safety of care. EBP allows clinicians and interprofessional teams to keep up with the rapidly changing environment.

The world is experiencing an information and technology explosion, and healthcare is no exception. Unfortunately, in healthcare, the growth of knowledge outpaces the application to practice. The process of incorporating new knowledge into clinical practice is often considerably delayed. Curry (2018) reports that it may take up to 15 years to approve new drugs. The average time for the uptake of research into actual practice is 17 years (Hanney et al., 2015). New knowledge has grown exponentially. Early in the 20th century, many healthcare professionals had but a few, hard-to-access journals available to them. Today, MEDLINE indexes 5,600 journals (National Library of Medicine, 2020), with more than 26 million references. The Cumulative Index to Nursing and Allied Health Literature (CINAHL) indexes more than 5,500 journals and includes more than 3.4 million records (EBSCO Publishing, 2020). Accessibility of information on the web also has increased consumer expectation of participating in treatment decisions. Patients with chronic health problems have accumulated considerable expertise in self-management, increasing the pressure for providers to be up to date with the best evidence for care.

Despite this knowledge explosion, healthcare clinicians can experience a decline in knowledge of best care practices that relates to the amount of information available and the limited time to digest it when no longer in a school or training environment. Estabrooks (1998) reported that knowledge of best care practices negatively correlated with year of graduation—that is, knowledge of best care practices declined as the number of years since graduation increased. EBP is one of the best strategies to enable healthcare providers to stay abreast of new practices and technology amid this continuing information explosion.

The objectives for this chapter are to:

- Define EBP
- Describe the evolution of EBP in healthcare
- Discuss EBP in relation to outcomes and accountability
- Highlight the healthcare clinician's role in EBP

EBP: Definition

EBP is a problem-solving approach to clinical decision-making within a healthcare organization. EBP integrates the best available scientific evidence with the best available experiential (patient and practitioner) evidence. EBP uses a deliberate approach to consider internal and external influences on practice and to encourage critical thinking in the judicious application of such evidence to the care of individual patients, a patient population, or a system (Dang & Dearholt, 2018). The challenge for healthcare providers is to use such evidence to implement the best interventions to improve patient outcomes. The Johns Hopkins Evidence-Based Practice Model (JHEBP) for Nursing and Healthcare Professionals provides a structured and systematic way for clinicians to effectively use current research and nonresearch evidence to determine best practices and provide safe, high-quality care.

EBP supports and informs clinical, administrative, and educational decision-making. Combining research, organizational experience (including quality improvement and financial data), clinical expertise, expert opinion, and patient preferences ensures clinical decisions based on all available evidence. EBP enhances efficacy (the ability to reach a desired result); efficiency (the achievement of a desired result with minimum expense, time, and effort); and effectiveness (the ability to produce a desired result). Additionally, EBP weighs risk, benefit, and cost against a backdrop of patient preferences. This evidence-based decision-making encourages healthcare providers to question practice and determine which interventions are ready to be implemented in clinical practice. EBP can lead to:

- Optimal outcomes
- Reductions in unnecessary variations in care
- Standardization of care
- Equivalent care at lower cost or in less time
- Improved patient satisfaction
- Increased clinician satisfaction and autonomy
- Higher health-related quality of life

The History

EBP in healthcare is not conceptually new. From a nursing perspective, Florence Nightingale pioneered the concept of using research evidence to dictate care (Nightingale, 1858). In the 1920s, Mary McMillan worked to bring a scientific basis to the practice of physical therapy and to standardize the practice (American Physical Therapy Association, 2020). As with any applied science, the terms associated with evidence-based practice changed as the science evolved. As early as 1972, Archibald L. Cochrane, a British medical researcher, criticized the health profession for administering treatments not supported by evidence (Cochrane, 1972). By the 1980s, the term evidence-based medicine was being used at McMaster University Medical School in Canada. Positive reception given to systematic reviews of care during pregnancy and childbirth prompted the British National Health Service in 1992 to approve funding for "a Cochrane Centre" to facilitate the preparation of systematic reviews of randomized controlled trials of healthcare, eventually leading to the establishment of the Cochrane Collaboration in 1993 (Cochrane Collaboration, 2016). Cochrane continues to provide systematic reviews about the effectiveness of healthcare and sound scientific evidence for providing effective treatment regimes. In 1996, Alan Pearson founded the Joanna Briggs Research Institute (now JBI) to link research with practice, thus impacting global health outcomes and providing evidence to inform clinical decision-making (JBI, 2020).

The use of tradition and ritual was and still is the basis for care by many clinicians. To use research in clinical practice, many disciplines sought scientific backing for common practices. For example, the Conduct and Utilization of Research in Nursing Project (CURN) (Horsley et al., 1978) aimed to develop and test a model for bringing research knowledge into clinical practice. Through the initial work, ten areas were identified as having adequate evidence to use in practice, and the authors published guidelines and nursing protocols for each area (Horsley et al., 1983):

- Structured preoperative teaching
- Reduction of diarrhea in tube-fed patients

- Preoperative sensory preparation to promote recovery
- Prevention of decubitus ulcers
- Intravenous cannula change
- Closed urinary drainage systems
- Distress reduction through sensory preparation
- Mutual goal-setting in patient care
- Clean intermittent catheterization
- Deliberate nursing interventions to reduce pain

This is just one example of many to highlight the beginning of using research in practice. However, EBP incorporates more than research findings. Clinician experience, patient preference, and internal organizational data are all used as evidence to inform decisions and improve patient outcomes. Building on these early efforts, EBP has evolved to include increasingly sophisticated analytical techniques; improved presentation and dissemination of information; advanced tools for searching and tracking literature; growing knowledge of how to implement findings while effectively considering patient preferences, costs, and policy issues; and a better understanding of how to measure effect and use feedback to promote ongoing improvement.

The Push for EBP

EBP has experienced tremendous growth in the past few decades. For example, the first detailed description of EBP and nursing in primary care was published in 1996; less than 10 years later, an entire journal dedicated to EBP, *Worldviews on Evidence-Based Nursing,* was published. This growth can be attributed to two main factors. First, as mentioned previously, knowledge development is outpacing our ability to put findings into practice, driving the need for a systematic way of evaluating evidence. Second, the development of EBP has been further driven by a desire to improve outcomes, pressure from consumers for more accountability, and regulatory requirements by accreditation bodies.

EBP and Outcomes

Healthcare providers, by nature, have always been interested in the outcomes and results of patient care. Traditionally, such results have been characterized in terms of morbidity and mortality. Recently, however, the focus has broadened to include clinical outcomes (e.g., hospital-acquired infection, falls, pressure ulcers), functional outcomes (e.g., performance of daily activities), quality-of-life outcomes (e.g., physical and mental health), and economic outcomes (e.g., direct, indirect, and intangible costs). EBP is an explicit process by which clinicians conduct critical evidence reviews and examine the link between healthcare practices and outcomes to inform decisions and improve the quality of care and patient safety.

EBP and Accountability

Nowhere is accountability a more sensitive topic than in healthcare. Knowing that patient outcomes are linked to evidence-based interventions is critical for promoting quality patient care. Professional and regulatory organizations and third-party payers mandate the use of evidence-based practices. Additionally, patients and families expect care to be based in best evidence. Public expectations that healthcare investments lead to high-quality results most likely will not diminish soon. In today's environment, quality and cost concerns drive healthcare. Consumers expect professionals to deliver the best evidence-based care with the least amount of risk.

Despite these mandates, much of the available data suggests that consumers are not consistently receiving appropriate care (IOM, 2001). Nurses and other healthcare professionals operate within an age of accountability (Leonenko & Drach-Zahavy, 2016); this accountability has become a focal point for healthcare (Pronovost, 2010). It is within this environment that nurses, physicians, public health scientists, and others explore what works and what does not. It is within this context that nurses and other healthcare providers continue the journey to bridge research and practice.

Governments and society challenge healthcare providers to base their practices on current, validated interventions. In 2012, the National Center for Advancing Translational Sciences at the National Institutes of Health was established to accelerate the translation of scientific discoveries into practice (Austin, 2016). Nursing has responded to the groundswell of information by educating nurses at every level to be competent practitioners of EBP and to close the gap between research and practice (Melnyk et al., 2017).

EBP provides a systematic approach to decision-making that leads to best practices and demonstrates clinician accountability for the care they provide. When the strongest available evidence is considered, the odds of doing the right thing at the right time for the right patient are improved. Given the complexity of linking research and clinical practice, EBP provides the most useful framework to translate evidence into practice.

The Healthcare Clinician's Role in EBP

EBP encompasses multiple sources of knowledge, clinical expertise, and patient preference. Because of their unique positions and expertise, nurses and other healthcare providers often play a pivotal role in generating questions about patient care and safety. This, along with the fact that practice questions and concerns often cross disciplines, makes it critical to enlist an interprofessional team and to include patient and family input as part of the process. Thus, clinicians need to develop the necessary knowledge and skills to not only participate in the EBP process but also serve as leaders of interdisciplinary teams seeking best practices to improve patient care. These leaders also play a vital role in modeling and promoting a culture that supports the use of collaborative EBP within the organization and in ensuring that the necessary resources (e.g., time, education, equipment, mentors, and library support) are in place to facilitate and sustain the process. The JHEBP model is an effective and efficient process for conducting EBP. The model has been used in many institutions and has been embraced by frontline nurses, pharmacists, occupational therapists, and many other disciplines. The tools developed as part of the model enable the team to use a step-by-step process for successfully completing an EBP project.

Summary

This chapter defines EBP and discusses the evolution that led to the critical need for practice based on evidence to guide decision-making. EBP creates a culture of critical thinking and ongoing learning and is the foundation for an environment in which evidence supports clinical and operational decisions, and decisions related to improvements in learning. EBP supports rational decision-making, reducing inappropriate variation in practice and making it easier for clinicians to do their job. EBP is an explicit process that facilitates meeting the needs of patients and delivering care that is effective, efficient, equitable, patient-centered, safe, and timely (IOM, 2001).

References

American Physical Therapy Association. (2020). *100 milestones of physical therapy*. https://centennial.apta.org/home/timeline/

Austin, C. P. (2016). *2016 director's messages*. National Center for Advancing Translational Sciences. https://ncats.nih.gov/director/message2016

Cochrane, A. L. (1972). *Effectiveness and efficiency: Random reflections on health services*. Nuffield Provincial Hospitals Trust.

Cochrane Collaboration. (2016). *About Cochrane*. http://www.cochrane.org/about-us

Curry, S. H. (2018). Translational science: Past, present, and future. *BioTechniques, 44*(2S). https://doi.org/10.2144/000112749

Dang, D., & Dearholt, S. (2012). *Johns Hopkins Nursing evidence-based practice: Model and guidelines* (2nd ed.). Sigma Theta Tau International.

EBSCO Publishing. (2020). *CINAHL Plus Full Text*. https://www.ebsco.com/products/research-databases/cinahl-plus-full-text

Estabrooks, C. A. (1998). Will evidence-based nursing practice make practice perfect? *Canadian Journal of Nursing Research, 30*(1), 15–36.

Hanney, S. R., Castle-Clarke, S., Grant, J., Guthrie, S., Henshall, C., Mestre-Ferrandiz, J., Pistollato, M., Pollitt, A., Sussex, J., & Wooding, S. (2015). How long does biomedical research take? Studying the time taken between biomedical and health research and its translation into products, policy, and practice. *Health Research Policy and Systems, 13*(1). https://doi.org/10.1186/1478-4505-13-1

Horsley, J., Crane, J., & Bingle, J. (1978). Research utilization as an organizational process. *Journal of Nursing Administration, 8*(7), 4–6. https://doi.org/10.1097/00005110-197807000-00001

Horsley, J. A., Crane, J., Crabtree, M. K., & Wood, D. J. (1983). *Using research to improve nursing practice*. Grune & Stratton.

Institute of Medicine. (2001). *Crossing the quality chasm: A new health system for the 21st century.* The National Academies Press.

Institute of Medicine. (2003). *Health professions education: A bridge to quality.* The National Academies Press.

JBI. (2020). *Our history.* https://joannabriggs.org/our-history

Leonenko, M., & Drach-Zahavy, A. (2016). "You are either out on the court, or sitting on the bench": Understanding accountability from the perspectives of nurses and nursing managers. *Journal of Advanced Nursing, 72*(11), 2718–2727. https://doi.org/10.1111/jan.13047

Melnyk, B. M., Gallagher-Ford, L., Long, L. E., & Fineout-Overholt, E. (2017). *Implementing the evidence-based practice (EBP) competencies in healthcare.* Sigma Theta Tau International.

National Library of Medicine. (2020). *MEDLINE: Overview.* https://www.nlm.nih.gov/bsd/medline.html

Nightingale, F. (1858). *Notes on matters affecting the health, efficiency, and hospital administration of the British Army.* Harrison & Sons. https://wellcomelibrary.org/item/b20387118#?c=0&m=0&s=0&cv=88&z=-1.2809%2C-0.0462%2C3.5618%2C1.8022

Pronovost, P. J. (2010). Learning accountability for patient outcomes. *JAMA, 304*(2), 204–205. https://doi.org/10.1001/jama.2010.979

Creating a Supportive EBP Environment

Why be concerned about creating a supportive environment for evidence-based practice (EBP)? The most obvious answer is that new evidence is continually surfacing in nursing and medical environments. Practitioners must incorporate the tremendous amount of newly generated knowledge into their daily routines for their practices to be evidence-based, yet there is a continuing well-documented delay in implementing new knowledge into practice environments. The dynamic and competitive US healthcare environment requires healthcare practitioners who are accountable to provide efficient and effective care. This environment also mandates continuous improvement in care processes and outcomes. Healthcare, provided within the structure of a system or an organization, can either facilitate or inhibit the uptake of best evidence. EBP requires the creation of an environment that fosters lifelong learning to increase the use of evidence in practice.

Because of the emphasis on quality and safety, many healthcare organizations have created strategic initiatives for EBP. Current national pay-for-performance initiatives—both voluntary and mandatory—provide reimbursement to hospitals and practitioners for implementing healthcare practices supported with evidence. Consumer pressure and increased patient expectations place an even greater emphasis on this need for true evidence-based practice. In an often-cited study, McGlynn et al. (2003) reported that Americans receive only about 50% of the healthcare recommended by evidence. A 2018 study found that only 8% of American adults age 35 and older received all recommended high-priority clinical preventive services, based on recommendations by the U.S. Preventive Services Task Force and Advisory Committee on Immunization Practices (Borsky, 2018).

Even with the increased emphasis on EBP, the majority of hospitals and practitioners are not implementing the available evidence and guidelines for care in their practices (Lehane et al., 2019). This suggests an even greater imperative to build infrastructure that not only supports EBP but also infuses it into practice environments.

Founded in 1970 as the Institute of Medicine (IOM), the National Academy of Medicine (NAM) is one of three academies that make up the National Academies of Sciences, Engineering, and Medicine (the National Academies) in the United States. As part of a restructuring of the National Academies in 2015, the IOM became NAM. Four previous IOM reports have called for healthcare professionals to focus on evidence-based practice:

- *Crossing the Quality Chasm* (2001) called for the healthcare system to adopt six aims for improvement and 10 principles for redesign. The report recommended that healthcare decision-making be evidence-based to ensure that patients receive care based on the best scientific evidence available, and that the evidence is transparent to patients and their families to assist them in making informed decisions.

- *Health Professions Education: A Bridge to Quality* (2003) described five key competencies for health professionals: delivering patient-centered care, working as part of interprofessional teams, focusing on quality improvement, using information technology, and practicing evidence-based medicine.

- *Roundtable on Evidence-Based Medicine* (2009) brought medical researchers and clinicians together to set a goal that by the year 2020, 90% of clinical decisions would be supported by accurate, timely, and up-to-date clinical information, and reflect the best available evidence—a goal that, unfortunately, healthcare professionals did not met.
- *The Future of Nursing: Leading Change, Advancing Health* (2011) urged that schools of nursing ensure that nurses achieve competency in leadership, health policy, systems improvement, teamwork and collaboration, and research and evidence-based practice.

A new type of healthcare worker exists now: one educated to think critically and not to simply accept the status quo. Generation Y, otherwise referred to as millennials, and Generation Z (socialmarketing.org/archives/generations-xy-z-and-the-others) question current practices, and, "We've always done it that way" is no longer an acceptable response. They want evidence that what they are doing in the workplace is efficient and effective. These new generations are pushing the profession away from practice based on tradition and past practices that are unsupported by evidence. This push requires that evidence support all clinical, operational, and administrative decision-making.

This compelling need for EBP in the healthcare environment requires proper planning, development, and commitment. This chapter:

- Explains how to choose an EBP model for use in the organization
- Describes leadership strategies to cultivate EBP
- Explores how to create and facilitate a supportive EBP environment
- Describes how to overcome common implementation barriers
- Discusses how to sustain the change

Choosing an EBP Model

It is critically important to establish a standardized approach to EBP inquiry in the organization. A standardized approach and choosing a model assures the team that appropriate methods are used to search, critique, and synthesize evidence when considering a change or improvement in systems, processes, and practice. A standardized approach facilitates implementation of best practices both clinically and administratively; identifies and improves cost components of care; fosters outcomes improvement; and ensures success of the EBP initiative.

Any EBP model or framework being reviewed for adoption should be carefully evaluated for:

- Fit, feasibility, and acceptability of the model with the vision, mission, philosophy, and values of the organization
- Educational background, leadership, experience, and practice needs of staff
- Presence of any partnerships for the EBP initiative, such as with schools that provide education for health professionals or collaboration with other professions, such as medicine, pharmacy, or nutrition
- Culture and environment of the organization
- Availability and access to sources of evidence internal or external to the organization

The leadership team should appoint a group to champion the EBP process and review models using the characteristics in this list and other organizational agreed-on criteria. Criteria for model review may include identifying strengths and weaknesses, evaluating assumptions, verifying ease of use, ensuring applicability for all clinical situations, reviewing examples of use and dissemination, and securing recommendations of other users.

Creating and Facilitating a Supportive EBP Environment

Successful infusion of evidence-based practice throughout the organization must focus on four key strategies: ensuring committed organizational leadership, establishing the culture, building capacity, and creating sustainability.

Ensuring Committed Organizational Leadership

Choosing the appropriate model to guide the systematic adoption of EBP across health professions and the organization is important; however, research has consistently found that supportive leadership is an essential component of the healthcare context that influences the successful implementation and uptake of EBP. Leadership's role is to create a supportive environment, empower clinicians, and be responsive to the tenets of EBP (Välimäki et al., 2018; Warren et al., 2016).

Evidence indicates that committed leadership cultivates the organizational context, work culture, and practice environment; encourages a spirit of inquiry, and enhances EBP across the organization, which results in improved outcomes (Dang et al., 2015; Pittman et al., 2019; Shuman et al., 2020).

Frontline leaders, and nurse managers specifically, play a key role in organizational climates that foster and promote EBP implementation by supporting, encouraging, and engaging the staff to drive change (Aasekjær et al., 2016; Kueny et al., 2015).

When leaders are actively involved and frequently consulted, the success of implementation, sustainability, and a stable infrastructure are more likely. When there is a lack of leader engagement, the change-and-transition process is more reactive than proactive, and the infrastructure and sustainability over time is less certain. Greenhalgh et al. (2004) describe three styles for managing the transition, change, and adoption of an innovation such as EBP:

- Leaders "let it happen" by communicating a passive style where, for example, small pockets of staff may self-organize to explore and create their own process for engaging in EBP.
- Leaders "help it happen" when a formal group such as advanced practice clinicians, acting as change champions, have invested in and defined an approach to EBP and have to negotiate for support and resources to implement it. Still, the leader is pulled into the process by change rather than leading it.

- The "make it happen" approach is intentional, systematic, planned, and fully engages all leaders in the process to ensure adoption, spread, and sustainability.

The highest level of discipline-specific leaders' support and visibility is paramount. The staff must see behaviors to advance the goal of infusing, building, and sustaining an evidence-based practice environment.

The organization's senior leadership can support EBP efforts best by modeling the practice and ensuring that all administrative decision-making is evidence-based. For example, if the organization's leaders ask middle managers for evidence (both organizational data and the best available research and nonresearch evidence) to support important decisions in their areas of responsibility, it is more likely that staff at all levels will also question and require evidence for their practice decisions. Additionally, all organizational departments' clinical and administrative standards (policies, protocols, and procedures) need to reflect best evidence and source citations. For example, at Hopkins, the infection control department implemented a policy regarding the use of artificial fingernails. Nurse managers (NM) were challenged with how to hold staff accountable for this change in policy, and subsequently, the senior leaders convened a group of NMs to conduct an EBP project on this topic. As a result, these managers were then armed with the best evidence on the risks associated with use of artificial nails and had direct experience with the EBP process and how it can strengthen administrative practice. With such leadership examples and activities, verbal and nonverbal EBP language and behaviors becomes a part of everyday activities and establishes an evidence-based culture.

Finally, the leader can further model support for EBP by participating in EBP change activities. For example, if the plan is to offer EBP education to the management group, the senior leader can attend and introduce the session by discussing the organization's vision of EBP. The leader's presence demonstrates the commitment to EBP and its value to the organization. Participating also gives the senior leader an appreciation for the process, including the time and resource commitment necessary for the organization to move toward an evidence-based practice.

To move the evidence-based practice initiative forward, the organization's senior leadership must ensure that the appropriate infrastructure is available and supported. This organizational infrastructure consists of human and material resources and a receptive culture.

Establishing the Organizational Culture

Establishing a culture of practice based on evidence is a leadership-driven change that fundamentally challenges commonly held beliefs about practice. This transformational change in culture typically occurs over a period of three to five years. During this time, leadership action builds EBP into the values, beliefs, norms, language, and structure of the organization and caregiving units through a planned and systematic approach.

Schein (2004) defines organizational culture as "patterns of shared basic assumptions that were learned by a group as it solved its problems of external adaption and internal integration, that has worked well enough…to be taught to new members as the correct way to perceive, think, and feel in relationship to these problems" (p. 17).

Thus, culture—a potent force operating below the surface—guides, constrains, or stabilizes the behavior of group members through shared group norms (Schein, 2004). Although organizations develop distinct cultures, subcultures also operate at the unit or team level and create a context for practice. Embedding a culture based on evidence requires that leaders at all levels explicitly challenge tradition, set expectations, model the use of evidence as the basis for decisions, and hold all levels of staff accountable for these behaviors.

The visible and tangible work of establishing a culture supportive of EBP requires revisiting the vision for use of best evidence in practice, the EBP strategic plan, identifying and exploiting the use of mentors and informal leaders, and overcoming barriers.

A tangible way to signal a change to a culture of evidence-based practice and lay the foundation for leadership commitment is in a clear and specific mission statement. This statement should include three key points:

- Speak to the spirit of inquiry and the lifelong learning necessary for evidence-based practice
- Address a work environment that demands and supports the healthcare team members' accountability for practice and decision-making
- Include the goal of improving patient care outcomes through evidence-based clinical, operational, and administrative decision-making

See Box 2.1 for an example of a mission statement from The Johns Hopkins Hospital (JHH) department of nursing. At JHH, the vice president of nursing and the directors wanted to ensure that the revisions in the mission resonated with and had meaning for the staff. After revising the document, they hosted an open forum with staff selected from all levels in the nursing department to provide input and feedback on the philosophy. This process highlighted the importance of this change, communicating leader commitment to EBP and to the part that staff would have in this change and transition.

Box 2.1 Excerpts From The Johns Hopkins Hospital Department of Nursing Mission

At The Johns Hopkins Hospital, we integrate the science of nursing, clinical knowledge, nursing judgment, and passionate commitment to quality care with the art of nursing, honoring patients' trust that they will be cared for with integrity and compassion.

In our practice…

- we are experts in the specialized treatment of illnesses;
- we pursue quality outcomes, advocating in the best interest of our patients;
- we embrace the responsibility of autonomous practice and commit to a collaborative approach to patient care;
- we seek, appraise, and incorporate the best evidence to support our practice;
- we master the application of healthcare technology;

Developing a Strategic Plan

Supportive and committed executive-level leadership must be involved in the creation and development of an evidence-based practice environment. To operationalize the vision and mission statements and build capacity for implementation of EBP, the organization's leaders must develop a strategic plan to identify goals and objectives, time frames, responsibilities, and an evaluation process. The plan also requires a commitment to allocate adequate resources to the EBP initiative, including people, time, money, education, and mentoring. Leaders should implement a strategic goal for evidence-based practice at all levels of the organization. As the initiative rolls out, leaders need to check the pulse of the organization and be prepared to modify the strategy as necessary. They should identify potential barriers to implementation, have a plan to reduce or remove them, and support the project directors and change champions in every way possible. Figure 2.1 outlines the essential elements of a strategic plan for initial implementation of EBP. As EBP develops over time, the content of the strategic plan should reflect the maturation of the program.

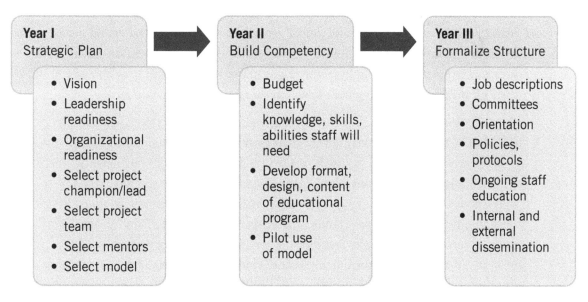

Figure 2.1 Elements of a strategic plan.

Identifying and Developing Mentors and Informal Leaders

Mentors and change champions have an important role in assimilation of EBP into the organizational culture. They provide a safe and supportive environment for staff to move out of their comfort zone as they learn new skills and competencies. Informal leaders influence the staff at the unit or departmental level. The presence and influence of both roles is a key attribute for sustainability and building capacity within staff. Because EBP is a leadership-driven change, leaders should identify and involve both formal and informal leaders early and often in creating the change and transition strategies so that they can serve as advocates rather than opponents for the change and model its use in practice.

Leadership must identify and select mentors with care, choosing them from across the organization—different roles, levels, and specialties. Consider who within the organization has the knowledge and skills to move an EBP initiative forward, can offer the best support, and has the most at stake to see that EBP is successful. When building the skills and knowledge of mentors, consider such questions as, "How will the mentors be trained? Who will provide the initial training? How and by whom will they be supported after their training is complete?" As the activities to build an EBP environment increase, leadership needs to diffuse education and mentoring activities throughout the staff. The key to success is to increase buy-in by involving as many staff as possible to champion the EBP process by focusing on a problem that is important to them.

Organizations can develop mentors in many ways. Initially, if the organization has not yet developed experts within their staff, it can find mentors through collaborative opportunities outside of the organization, such as partnerships with schools or consultation with organizations and experts who have developed models. After internal expertise is established, the implementation of EBP throughout the organization results in a self-generating mechanism for developing mentors. For example, members of committees who participate in EBP projects guided by a mentor quickly become mentors to other staff, committees, or groups who are engaged in EBP work. EBP fellowships are another way to develop mentors; the fellow gains skills to lead and consult with staff groups within their home department or throughout the organization.

Evidence indicates that, when facing a clinical concern, clinicians prefer to ask a colleague rather than search a journal, book, or the internet for the answer. Colleagues sought out are often informal leaders, and evidence indicates that these informal leaders—opinion leaders and change champions—are effective in changing teams' behaviors if used in combination with education and performance feedback (Titler, 2008). Formal leaders differ from informal leaders in that formal leaders have position power, whereas informal leaders' power is derived from their status, expertise, and opinions within a group.

Opinion leaders are the go-to persons with a wide sphere of influence whom peers would send to represent them, and they are "viewed as a respected source of influence, considered by [peers] as technically competent, and trusted to judge the fit between the innovation [EBP] and the local [unit] situation. …[O]pinion leaders' use of the innovation [EBP] influences peers and alters group norms" (Titler, 2008, pp. 1–18). Change champions have a similar impact, but they differ in that although they practice on the unit, they are not part of the unit staff. They circulate information, encourage peers to adopt the innovation, orient staff to innovations, and are persistent and passionate about the innovation (Titler, 2008).

The identification of champions can occur at two levels. The first is at the organizational level. These include, for example, clinical specialists, advance practice providers, and departmental subject matter experts as change champions. The second group of champions is at the departmental level and includes departmental members whom the staff view as role models for professional practice and who can hold staff accountable. They are clinicians committed to clinical inquiry and, many times, are initially identified because of their interest in the topic or issue for an EBP project or because they are skillful collaborators and team players.

The critical role of mentors and informal leaders in facilitating EBP and translating the evidence into practice has been the focus of significant work (Dearholt et al., 2008; Titler, 2008). Mentoring and facilitation are needed throughout the EBP process to help healthcare team members be successful and to promote excellence (Bisset et al., 2016).

Overcoming Barriers to Fostering EBP Culture

One ongoing responsibility of leadership is to identify and develop a plan to overcome barriers to the implementation and maintenance of an EBP environment. Leaders must not underestimate this responsibility and must be a visible part of the implementation plan.

Those involved in EBP have repeatedly cited time constraints as a barrier that prevents implementation of EBP and the continued use of an inquiry model for practice. Providing clinical release time to staff participating in an EBP project is essential. Experience shows that staff need time to think about and discuss the EBP project; to read the latest evidence; and to appraise the strength (level and quality) of that evidence. Reading research and critiquing evidence is challenging and demanding work for clinicians and requires blocks of time set aside. EBP, an essential professional responsibility, cannot be done in stolen moments away from patients or in brief, 15-minute intervals. Healthcare team members require uninterrupted time away from the clinical unit.

A *lack of supportive leadership* for EBP is another major barrier to the creation and maintenance of an EBP environment. Senior leaders must incorporate EBP into their roles and normative behavior. To create a culture of organizational support for EBP, the day-to-day language must be consistent with using evidence and be a part of the organizational values. That is, leaders must talk the talk—making a point to ask, "Where is the evidence?" Leaders must also walk the walk, demonstrating daily a regard for evidence in their actions and behaviors. Does the organization value science and research and hold its staff accountable for using the best evidence in practice and clinical decision-making? Do leaders expect that routine decisions be based on the best possible data and evidence, or do practitioners default to experience or history, financial restrictions, or even emotion? Do leaders themselves use the best evidence available for administrative decision-making? Does the organizational chart reflect a leader for departments such as research and quality improvement? To whom do they report? Are these roles centralized or decentralized in the organizational structure?

A *lack of organizational infrastructure* to support EBP is another significant barrier. Resources—in terms of people, money, and time—require negotiation and allocation to support the initiative. Staff must be able to access library resources, computers, and current evidence in online database resources. Experts, such as the champions and mentors, must also be part of the available infrastructure.

Healthcare team members themselves can be a significant barrier to implementing EBP. They often lack the skills, knowledge, and confidence to read results of research studies and translate them into practice. Some also may resist EBP through negative attitudes and skepticism toward research. In some organizations, staff may feel they have limited authority to make or change practice decisions and are skeptical that anything can result from the pursuit of evidence. Another potential barrier is the nature of the interprofessional relationships among disciplines, specialists, subject matter experts, and physicians.

Lack of communication is a common barrier to implementation of any change but is particularly detrimental to EBP initiatives. To overcome this barrier, EBP teams can design a communication plan for an EBP initiative. As the staff develops EBP and approaches the clinical environment with critical thinking, they want to know that what they are doing is valued. The staff expects leaders to be responsive and open to their concerns or questions during implementation of the change. Staff will take ownership of the change if they sense that their leaders are partners in the change process.

A final barrier is *lack of incentives, recognition, or rewards* in the organization for engaging in EBP projects. Leaders should assess whether the organization's systems nurture or limit EBP work and whether an accountability-based environment exists. Establishing an EBP environment and continuing EBP project work is challenging and requires a level of commitment on the part of all involved. The leadership team should understand the need for—and include incentives to foster—meaningful work and professional development of staff as part of the EBP implementation process. These are crucial discussion points during the planning, implementation, and maintenance of the change. Barriers are best dealt with through prevention and planning to assess and identify staff needs.

Leading Culture Change and Managing Transition

A key factor for success when undergoing a culture change is that leaders and those assigned to implement the change understand the difference between change and transition (see Table 2.1) and how to lead change and manage transitions (Bridges & Bridges, 2017); this understanding provides insights on how to overcome the barriers discussed earlier.

Table 2.1 Definitions of Change and Transition

Change	An event that has a defined start and ending point and occurs external to us
Transition	An emotional or psychological process that occurs internally—inside the hearts and minds of staff as they come to grips with the new way of doing things

Change is an event that has clear and tangible start and stop points. For example, a staff-led EBP project finds that patients and families prefer clinical staff to wear color-coded scrub wear to distinguish among team members. Based on this evidence, leaders decide to change to standard colors for scrub wear for all clinical staff. This is change—it begins with selecting colors for clinicians and ends when staff begin wearing the new scrubs. Transition, on the other hand, involves "letting go" of something familiar, valued, or treasured, which generates a feeling of loss. When staff are labeled "resistant to change," it is more accurately the transition they are resisting—the emotional process. Though change can take place in a short period, the time trajectory for transitions is different for each person and defined by their emotional state at any given moment. Therefore, to understand why some staff may resist change, leaders of the change have to understand what staff will have to let go of when standardizing scrub wear.

The scope and complexity of the change and the amount of spread determines the amount of planning for change and transition. Some changes may consist of simple, straightforward communication or educational "fast facts" on a device such as switching from use of a flutter valve to an incentive spirometer on a post-operative surgical unit. On the other hand, the change may be complex, multifaceted, and hospital-wide, such as implementation of a nurse-managed heparin protocol that affects nurse and physician responsibilities and workflow across the hospital. In either situation, knowing the difference between change and transition is important to success.

Strategies for Managing Transitions

Strategies for managing change are concrete and guided by tactical project plans such as those outlined in Appendix A. However, when change activities spark resistance, it is a clue that the staff are dealing with transition—the human side of the change. Resistance to change is how feelings of loss manifest, and these are not always concrete. Losses may be related to attitudes, expectations, assumptions—all of which make up staff comfort zones and provide them with a sense of routine and familiarity in what they do every day.

One way to head off resistance is to talk with staff about what they feel they stand to lose in doing things a new way—in other words, assess their losses. Another strategy to help staff move through the transition is to describe the change in as much detail as possible and to be specific so that staff can form a clear picture of where the transition will lead, why the change is needed and results if the change is not made, and what part the staff play. In assessing loss, leaders need to think of individuals and groups that will be affected by the change both directly and downstream of the practice, system, or process that is being changed. Because transitions are subjective experiences, not all staff will perceive and express the same losses. Examples of the range of losses include competence, routines, relationships, status, power, meaning to their work, turf, group membership, and personal identity (Bridges & Bridges, 2017). Specific strategies to address these transitions include:

- Talk with staff openly to understand their perceptions of what is ending. Frontline clinicians have enormous wisdom, and what they see as problems with the change should be respected and tapped into by valuing rather than judging their dissent. Do this simply, directly, and with empathy. For example, say, "I see your hesitation in supporting the new scrub wear decision. Help me understand why." In the end, staff are likely to move through the transition more quickly if given the chance to talk openly about their losses.

- Because culture is local, tailor how the change is implemented to the context of the caregiving unit where staff work; staff need to own this action locally. This is one reason that informal leaders and change champions are important.

- Clarify what is staying the same to minimize overgeneralization and overreaction to the change.

- After acknowledging the loss, honor the past for what staff has accomplished. Present the change as a concept that builds on this past. One way to do this is with symbolic events or rituals that can be powerful markers of honoring the past. For example, staff may create a quilt or collage of pieces or patterns of their scrub wear or write on a large poster in the break room to mark what they are letting go.

- It is human nature for staff to complain first, before they accept the new way of doing things. Avoid arguing about the statements you hear, because it shuts down communication; rather, liberally use your active listening skills. Understanding is more important than agreement. Be transparent and let staff know when you do not know the answer; commit to finding out.

Change teams should not underestimate the significance of communication in the change-and-transition process. Communication is essential in building broad support at both the organizational and local levels. A key strategy is to be transparent and say everything more than once. Because of the amount of information staff receive, they need to hear it multiple times before they begin to pay attention. Bridges and Bridges (2017) recommends a rule of six times, six different ways, focused at the local level in explicit terms. For staff to see the outcome of the change and move through the transition, you need to follow these four communication guidelines:

1. Describe clearly where you are going with the change; if people understand what the purpose is, and the problem that led to the change, they will be better able to manage the uncertainty that comes with transition.

2. One outcome of communication is to leave staff with a clear, specific picture of what things will look like when the change is completed: What will the new workflow be? How will it look? What will it feel like? Who are the new players?

3. Explain the *plan* for change in as much detail as you have at the time; be transparent—if you don't know something, say so, and always follow with when, or what you will need, to answer their question at a later time.

4. People own what they create, so let staff know what you need from them, what part they will have, and where they will have choices or input.

Building Capacity

Building capacity refers to arming staff with the knowledge, skills, and resources to procure and judge the value of evidence and translate it into practice. EBP education and direct practice gained through work on interprofessional teams is the most effective strategy to build competency to use and apply EBP.

Developing EBP Knowledge and Skills

The most popular format for EBP education programs at Hopkins is the one-day workshop. The morning session covers EBP concepts, the JHEBP Model and Guidelines, and evidence searching and appraisal techniques. In the afternoon, attendees critique and appraise the evidence for an EBP question and decide, as a group, whether a practice change is warranted based on the evidence available to them. Hopkins experts have successfully implemented the one-day workshop in many settings outside of Hopkins, including in rural, community, and nonteaching hospitals and other large academic medical centers. Table 2.2 outlines the educational topics and objectives for the one-day workshop.

Table 2.2 One-Day Workshop Topics and Objectives

Subject Area	Objectives
Introduction to Evidence-Based Practice	Explain the origins of EBP Discuss the importance of EBP Define EBP
Guidelines for Implementation	Describe the JHEBP Model Discuss plans for using the model Explain the steps in the process Discuss how to develop an answerable question
Appraising Evidence	Describe the different levels of evidence Determine where to look for evidence
Searching for Evidence	Discuss library services: • How to have a search run by the library • How to order articles • How to do a basic literature search
Appraising the Evidence Application	Provide explanation of the evidence appraisal forms Facilitate group appraisal or evaluation of assigned articles Discuss level of appraisal and quality of each article Complete individual and overall evidence summary forms
Summarizing the Evidence and Beyond	Facilitate discussion of synthesis of the evidence Determine whether practice changes are indicated based on the evidence Describe fit, feasibility, and acceptability of practice change Discuss how the practice change can be implemented Discuss how changes can be evaluated

Access to Information and Library Services

Librarians' skills in searching, organizing, and evaluating information can contribute to furthering the development of EBP and creating a positive impact on interprofessional staff and patient outcomes (Marshall et al., 2013). Almost all of the respondents (95%) said the information found with the help of librarians resulted in better-informed clinical decisions. Findings from their study showed that the availability and use of library and information resources and services consistently affected how clinicians gave advice to patients, handled patient care problems (diagnoses, tests, treatments, medication errors), avoided adverse events, and saved time.

Over the last several decades, a number of researchers have conducted reviews of the literature to examine how healthcare professionals acquire and use information to inform practice (Davies & Harrison, 2007; Hurst & Mickan, 2017; Isham et al., 2016; Spenceley et al., 2008). Findings indicate that health professionals prefer face-to-face meetings, collegial discussion, and print materials over evidence-based resources. The preference for informal learning sources is in part a result of common barriers clinicians face, such as clinical demands, lack of availability of current resources and time, limited searching skills, and issues with online resources. If an organization provides easy access to resources for practice inquiry and creates an expectation of their use, EBP can flourish. Those who do not provide such resources must address this critical need.

The Johns Hopkins Evidence-Based Practice Model implementation team found that indicators of success of an environment supportive of inquiry included the following conditions:

- Staff has access to reference books and the internet on the patient care unit.
- Journals are available in hard copy or online.
- A medical and nursing library is available.
- Knowledgeable library personnel are available to support staff and assist with evidence searches.
- Other resources for inquiry and EBP are available.

Interprofessional Collaboration

In today's team-focused healthcare environment, interprofessional collaboration for the evaluation and dissemination of evidence in the healthcare work setting is a high priority because many practice changes involve all members of the healthcare team, administrators, and policymakers. A conference held in February 2011 in Washington, DC—sponsored by the Health Resources and Services Administration (HRSA), Josiah Macy Jr. Foundation, Robert Wood Johnson Foundation, ABIM Foundation, and Interprofessional Education Collaborative (IPEC)—brought together more than 80 leaders from various health professions to review "Core Competencies for Interprofessional Collaborative Practice" (IPEC Expert Panel, 2011). The meeting's agenda focused on creating action strategies for the core competencies to transform health professional education and healthcare delivery in the United States. Competency Domain 4 supported the need for interprofessional teams to provide evidence-based care: "Apply relationship-building values and the principles of team dynamics to perform effectively in different team roles to plan and deliver patient-/population-centered care that is safe, timely, efficient, effective, and equitable" (p. 25). When developing EBP teams, consider interprofessional participation and the identification and development of EBP mentors from all the health professions.

It is widely recognized that education to develop skills and knowledge about EBP is essential for today's healthcare professional (IOM, 2003). This education is important at all levels of education. The development of a collaboration with schools that prepare and educate health professionals is mutually reinforcing. The practice organization can provide real-life EBP questions for the students to use in their research courses. As a course assignment and using the questions provided by the collaborating school, students search and critique the available evidence to inform the practice question from free literature databases such as CINAHL Plus, Cochrane, Embase, PsycINFO, PubMed, and Web of Science. The students prepare a summary of the evidence, synthesize the findings, and make general recommendations for the practice organization to evaluate and consider translating to their practice.

EBP is an essential competency for all health professionals and is no longer optional (IOM, 2003). Programs require that students understand the EBP process and use results to generate new knowledge for the profession. The collaboration between or among disciplines provides a strong team approach to improve clinical practice. Practice questions, issues, and concerns are often generated at the point of care by frontline clinicians. These practice questions result in evidence search, critique, and synthesis of findings. However, when the synthesis of findings is not strong or clear, it requires further evaluation. This evaluation often involves a pilot study to generate new evidence. The involvement of PhD-prepared research healthcare practitioners is critical to the design of research and generation of new knowledge. This collaborative approach to practice between doctorate-prepared professions is the goal for practice organizations.

Finally, collaboration with health profession schools can also foster the creation of faculty practice arrangements and faculty development. The development of a faculty practice can take many shapes, including both direct and indirect practice collaborations, depending on the needs of the practice organization and the school. A collaboration can be beneficial for both groups by effectively integrating EBP concepts into curricula and for professional development in the organization.

Sustaining the Change

At the beginning of an EBP strategic initiative, the organization's leaders must support and sustain a change in how the organization approaches its work. The leaders, mentors, and change champions and those responsible for the initiative must continually listen to the staff and be responsive to their comments, questions, and concerns. For EBP to be fully adopted and integrated into the organization, staff must feel that changing practice will improve quality of care and make a difference in patients' lives. The passion will be palpable when EBP becomes a part of everyday practice. Therefore, sustaining the change requires an infrastructure that aligns staff expectations and organizational structures with the strategic vision and plan for a culture based on evidence.

Setting Expectations for EBP

Setting role expectations for EBP through development of job descriptions, orientation programs, and performance evaluation tools is a first step in developing human capital for EBP and for hardwiring the culture of practice based on evidence. These personnel tools should be developed or revised to emphasize the staff's responsibility and accountability for making administrative and practice decisions based on best evidence to improve patient care outcomes and processes. The tools must be consistent across the employment continuum. For example, job descriptions should state professional expectations in terms of everyday performance and measurement of competence. The orientation should introduce professionals to how the organization develops and evaluates competencies. The performance evaluation tool should measure the level of performance on the standards and competencies for EBP practice.

Committee Structure

Standing professional practice committees and their members take on the roles of EBP change champions and mentors. Each committee serves a different but important role for implementing EBP throughout the organization. Professional practice committee structures are designed to promote excellence in patient care, practice, education, and all forms of inquiry (EBP, quality improvement, research) by:

- Recruiting and retaining a diverse professional staff
- Establishing evidence-based standards of care and practice
- Promoting interprofessional inquiry
- Advancing professional growth and development

Table 2.3 describes EBP functions for the department of nursing professional practice committees.

Table 2.3 Department of Nursing Committee Functions Related to EBP

Committee	Functions
EBP Steering Committee	Establishes strategic initiatives for EBP within and external to Johns Hopkins Health System and Johns Hopkins University School of Nursing
Clinical Quality Improvement Committee	Promotes evidence-based improvements in systems and processes of care to achieve safe, high-quality patient outcomes
Leadership Development Committee	Recommends and implements innovative evidence-based strategies for management and leadership practice
Research Committee	Supports discovery of new knowledge and translation into nursing practice
Standards of Care Committee	Promotes, develops, and maintains evidence-based standards of care
Standards of Practice Committee	Promotes, develops, and maintains evidence-based standards of professional practice

Communication Plan

A communication plan should be an integral part of both the EBP process and its sustainability. The plan should address:

- The goals of the communication
- Target audiences
- Available communication media
- Preferred frequency
- Important messages

Minimally, the goals for an EBP communication plan should focus on staff to increase awareness of the initiative, educate staff regarding their contribution, highlight and celebrate successes, and inform staff about EBP activities throughout the organization. Consider developing an EBP website within the organization's intranet. This website can be an excellent vehicle for communicating EBP information, including questions under consideration, projects in progress or completed, outcomes, and available EBP educational opportunities. The website can also serve as a snapshot and history of an organization's EBP activities and can be helpful when seeking or maintaining Magnet designation.

Finally, the communication plan can use online surveys to involve staff by asking opinions about potential or completed work, maintaining a finger on the pulse of initiatives, and developing EBP "messages." Messages can target the communication, link the initiative to the organization's mission, and give a consistent vision while providing new and varied information about the initiative.

After movement toward a supportive EBP environment begins, the biggest challenge is to keep the momentum going. To sustain the change, the staff must own the change and work to sustain it in a practice environment that values critical thinking and uses evidence for all administrative and clinical decision-making.

When resources are allocated to an EBP initiative, some may raise questions about expenditures and the costs related to EBP. To sustain the work of and value to the organization, EBP project work needs to reflect and align with the organization's priorities. It is helpful to identify EBP projects that improve safety or solve risk management problems; address wide variations in practice or in clinical practice that are different from the community standard; or solve high-risk, high-volume, or high-cost problems. Consider asking these questions: "Is there evidence to support the organization's current practice? Are these the best achievable outcomes? Is there a way to be more efficient or cost-effective?" Improvements or benefits to the organization could result in any of these important areas if EPB work identified best practices to improve outcomes of care, decrease costs, or decrease risks associated with the problem. Sustaining the change also involves developing an evaluation plan to identify process and outcome performance measures that monitor implementation, commitment, and results.

The measures should determine the usefulness, satisfaction, and success of the EBP environment. Are the initiatives changing or supporting current practice? What best practices or exemplars have resulted? Has the organization saved money or become more efficient? What performance data shows that this is making a difference to the organization? The evaluation plan should include a timeline and triggers that would signal when a modification of the plan is necessary.

Summary

We have learned many lessons in the development, implementation, and continual refinement of the JHEBP Model and Guidelines. The need to create a supportive EBP environment is one of the most important lessons. Essential to that effort is recognition of the importance of capacity building for EBP. Supportive leaders' help at all levels is essential to establish a culture of EBP, including the expansion of infrastructure and the allocation of resources—such as time, money, and people—to sustain the change. Leaders set priorities, facilitate the process, and set expectations. The development of local mentors and champions contributes to the successful implementation of EBP and helps overcome barriers and resistance to EBP.

A culture of critical thinking and ongoing learning creates an environment where evidence supports clinical and administrative decisions, ensuring the highest quality of care by using evidence to promote optimal outcomes, reduce inappropriate variation in care, and promote patient and staff satisfaction. Working in an EBP environment changes the way healthcare team members think about and approach that work. As the staff develop expertise in the EBP process, their professional growth and engagement begins a personal and organizational trajectory leading to evidence-based decisions, a higher level of critical review of evidence, and engagement as valued contributors in the interprofessional team.

References

Aasekjær, K., Waehle, H. V., Ciliska, D., Nordtvedt, M. W., & Hjalmhult, E. (2016). Management involvement—A decisive condition when implementing evidence-based practice. *Worldviews on Evidence-Based Nursing, 13*(1), 32–41. https://doi.org/10.1111/wvn.12141

Bissett, K., Cvach, M., & White, K. (2016). Improving competence and confidence with evidence-based practice among nurses: Outcomes of a quality improvement project. *Journal for Nurses in Professional Development*, 32(5), 248–255. https://doi.org/10.1097/NND.0000000000000293

Borsky, A., Zhan, C., Miller, T., Ngo-Metzger, Q., Bierman, A., & Meyers, D. (2018). Few Americans receive all high-priority, appropriate clinical preventive services. *Health Affairs*, 37(6), 925–928. https://doi.org/10.1377/hlthaff.2017.1248

Bridges, W., & Bridges, S. M. (2017). *Managing transitions: Making the most of change* (4th ed.). Da Capo Press.

Dang, D., Melnyk, B., Fineout-Overholt, E., Ciliska, D., DiCenso, A., Cullen, L., & Stevens, K. (2015). Models to guide implementation and sustainability of evidence-based practice. In B. M. Melnyk & E. Fineout-Overholt (Eds), *Evidence-based practice in nursing and healthcare: A guide to best practice* (3rd ed.). Wolters-Kluwer Health.

Davies, K., & Harrison, J. (2007). The information seeking behavior of doctors: A review of the evidence. *Health Information Library Journal*, 24(2), 78–94. https://doi.org/10.1111/j.1471-1842.2007.00713.x

Dearholt, S. L., White, K. M., Newhouse, R., Pugh, L. C., & Poe, S. (2008). Educational strategies to develop evidence-based practice mentors. *Journal for Nurses in Staff Development*, 24(2), 53–59. https://doi.org/10.1097/01.NND.0000300873.20986.97

Greenhalgh, T., Robert, G., Macfarlane, F., Bate, P., & Kyriakidou, O. (2004). Diffusion of innovations in service organizations: Systematic review and recommendations. *The Milbank Quarterly*, 82(4), 581–629. https://onlinelibrary.wiley.com/doi/full/10.1111/j.0887-378X.2004.00325.x

Hurst, D., & Mickan, S. (2017). Describing knowledge encounters in healthcare: A mixed studies systematic review and development of a classification. *Implementation Science*, 12(35), 2–14.

Institute of Medicine (US) Committee on Quality of Health Care in America. (2001). *Crossing the quality chasm: A new health system for the 21st century*. National Academies Press.

Institute of Medicine Committee on the Health Professions Education Summit. (2003). A. C. Greiner & E. Knebel (Eds.), *Health professions education: A bridge to quality*. National Academies Press.

Institute of Medicine. (2009). *Roundtable on evidence-based medicine*. National Academies Press. https://www.ncbi.nlm.nih.gov/books/NBK52847/

Institute of Medicine Committee on the Robert Wood Johnson Foundation Initiative on the Future of Nursing, at the Institute of Medicine. (2011). *The future of nursing: Leading change, advancing health*. National Academies Press.

Interprofessional Education Collaborative Expert Panel. (2011). *Core competencies for interprofessional collaborative practice: Report of an expert panel*. Interprofessional Education Collaborative.

Isham, A., Bettiol, I. A., Hoang. H., & Crocombe, L. (2016). A systematic literature review of the information-seeking behavior of dentists in developed countries. *Journal of Dental Education*, 80(5), 569–577.

Kueny, A., Shever, L. L., Mackin, M. L., & Titler, M. G. (2015). Facilitating the implementation of evidence-based practice through contextual support and nursing leadership. *Journal of Healthcare Leadership*, 7, 29–39. https://doi.org/10.2147/JHL.S45077

Lehane, E., Leahy-Warren, P., O'Riordan, C., Savage, E., Drennan, J., O'Tuathaigh, C., O'Connor, M., Corrigan, M., Burke, F., Hayes, M., Lynch, H., Sahm, L., Heffernan, E., O'Keeffe, E., Blake, C., Horgan, F., & Hegarty, J. (2019). Evidence-based practice education for healthcare professions: An expert view. *BMJ Evidence-Based Medicine, 24*(3), 103–108. https://doi.org/10.1136/bmjebm-2018-111019

Marshall, J. G., Sollenberger, J., Easterby-Gannett, S., Morgan, L. K., Klem, M. L., Cavanaugh, S. K., Oliver, K. B., Thompson, C. A., Romanosky, N., & Hunter, S. (2013). The value of library and information services in patient care: Results of a multisite study. *Journal of Medical Library Association, 101*(1), 38–46. https://doi.org/10.3163/1536-5050.101.1.007

McGlynn, E. A., Asch, S. M., Adams, J., Keesey, J., Hicks, J., DeCristofaro, A., & Kerr, E. A. (2003). The quality of health care delivered to adults in the United States. *New England Journal of Medicine, 348*(26), 2635–2645. https://doi.org/10.1056/NEJMsa022615

Pittman, J., Cohee, A., Storet, S., LaMothe, J., Gilbert, J., Bakoyannis, G., Ofner, S., & Newhouse, R. (2019). A multisite health system survey to assess organizational context to support evidence-based practice. *Worldviews on Evidence-Based Nursing, 16*(4), 271–280. https://doi.org/10.1111/wvn.12375

Schein, E. H. (2004). *Organizational culture and leadership* (3rd ed.). Jossey-Bass.

Shuman, C. J., Ehrhart, M. G., Torres, E. M., Veliz, P., Kath, L. M., VanAntwerp, K., . . . Aarons, G. A. (2020). EBP implementation leadership of frontline nurse managers: Validation of the Implementation Leadership Scale in acute care. *Worldviews on Evidence-Based Nursing, 17*(1), 82–91.

Spenceley, S. M., O'Leary, K. A., Chizawsky, L. L. K., Ross, A. J., & Estabrooks, C. A. (2008). Sources of information used by nurses to inform practice: An integrative review. *International Journal of Nursing Studies, 45*(6), 954–70. https://doi.org/10.1016/j.ijnurstu.2007.06.003

Titler, M. G. (2008). The evidence for evidence-based practice implementation. In R. G. Hughes (Ed.), *Patient safety and quality: An evidence-based handbook for nurses.* AHRQ Publication No. 08-0043. Agency for Healthcare Research and Quality.

Välimäki, T., Partanen, P., & Häggman-Laitila, A. (2018). An integrative review of interventions for enhancing leadership in the implementation of evidence-based nursing. *Worldviews on Evidence-Based Nursing, 15*(6), 424–431. https://doi.org/10.1111/wvn.12331

Warren, J. I, McLaughlin, M., Bardsley, J., Eich, J., Esche, C. A., Kropkowski, L., & Risch, S. (2016). The strengths and challenges of implementing EBP in healthcare systems. *Worldviews on Evidence-Based Nursing, 13*(1), 15–24. https://doi.org/10.1111/wvn.12149

The Johns Hopkins Evidence-Based Practice Model and Guidelines

3 The Johns Hopkins Evidence-Based Practice (JHEBP) Model for Nurses and Healthcare Professionals (HCPs) Process Overview 43

The Johns Hopkins Evidence-Based Practice (JHEBP) Model for Nurses and Healthcare Professionals (HCPs) Process Overview

Evidence-based practice (EBP) is a core competency for all healthcare professionals (HCPs) in all practice settings (Saunders et al., 2019). Using an evidence-based approach to care and practice decision-making is not only an expectation in all practice settings, but also a requirement established by professional standards, regulatory agencies, health insurers, and purchasers of healthcare insurance. EBP is an important component of high reliability organizations and is a process that can enable organizations to meet the quadruple healthcare aim to enhance patient care, improve population health, reduce healthcare costs, and increase the well-being of healthcare staff (Migliore et al., 2020).

In 2009, the Institute of Medicine (IOM) set an ambitious goal that 90% of clinical decisions would be evidence-based by 2020. Although healthcare professionals are increasingly adopting EBP in practice, we have not met this grand challenge. However, licensed healthcare staff have the potential to make a major impact to improve patient outcomes through the appraisal and translation of evidence

(American Association of Colleges of Nursing [AACN, 2020; IOM, 2011; Wilson et al., 2015). This requires leaders in both academia and service settings to align their learning and practice environments to promote evidence-based healthcare, to cultivate a spirit of continuous inquiry, and to translate the highest-quality evidence into practice. Using a model for EBP within an organization fosters end-user adoption of evidence, enables users to speak a common language, standardizes processes, improves care and care outcomes, and embeds this practice into the fabric of the organization. The objectives for this chapter are to:

- Describe the revised Johns Hopkins Evidence-Based Practice Model for Nurses and Healthcare Professionals (HCPs)
- Introduce frontline HCPs and leaders to the PET process (Practice Question, Evidence, and Translation)

The Johns Hopkins Evidence-Based Practice (JHEBP) Model for Nurses and HCPs—Essential Components: Inquiry, Practice, and Learning

The revised Johns Hopkins Evidence-Based Practice (JHEBP) Model for Nurses and HCPs (see Figure 3.1) is composed of three interrelated components—inquiry, practice, and learning—that take place in the context of interprofessional collaborative practice.

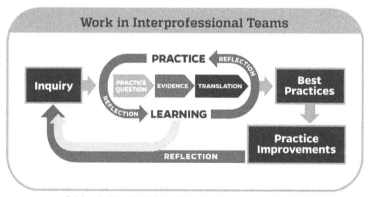

© Johns Hopkins Health System/Johns Hopkins University School of Nursing

Figure 3.1 The Johns Hopkins Evidence-Based Practice Model for Nurses and HCPs (2020).

Inquiry

In the revised JHEBP Model, inquiry is the initial component that launches the EBP process. The concept of *inquiry*, a foundation for healthcare practice, encompasses a focused effort to question, examine, and collect information about a problem, an issue, or a concern generally identified through observation, assessment, and personal experience within the clinical setting. Curiosity and inquiry can foster meaningful learning experiences by prompting individuals to look for learning opportunities to know more. The National League for Nursing (NLN; 2014) describes a spirit of inquiry as

> *a persistent sense of curiosity that informs both learning and practice. A nurse infused by a spirit of inquiry will raise questions, challenge traditional and existing practices, and seek creative approaches to problem-solving. ...A spirit of inquiry...engenders innovative thinking and extends possibilities for discovering novel solutions in both predictable and unpredictable situations* (NLN, 2014, para. 1).

Within the practice setting, inquisitiveness and curiosity about the best evidence to guide clinical decision-making drive EBP (Melnyk et al., 2009). Questions about practice commonly arise from HCPs as they provide everyday care to their patients. These questions may include whether best evidence is being used or if the care provided is safe, effective, timely, accessible, cost-effective, and of high quality. Organizations that foster a culture of inquiry are more likely to have staff that will embrace and actively participate in EBP activities (Migliore et al., 2020). When HCPs, individually and collectively, commit to inquiry and apply new knowledge and best evidence in practice, two outcomes are more likely—high-quality outcomes and a culture that promotes inquiry.

Practice

Practice, one component of all HCPs' activity, reflects the translation of what clinicians know into what they do. As with all health professions, it is the who, what, when, where, why, and how that addresses the range of activities that define the care a patient receives (American Nurses Association [ANA], 2010, 2015).

All HCPs are bound by and held to standards established by their respective professional organizations. For example, the ANA (2015) has identified six standards of nursing practice (scope) that are based on the nursing process and 11 standards of professional performance. In addition to the ANA, professional nursing specialty organizations establish standards of care for specific patient populations. Collectively, these standards define nurses' scope of practice, set expectations for evaluating performance, and guide the care provided to patients and families. Similarly, other HCP organizations establish practice standards for a variety of care providers, such as the American College of Clinical Pharmacy's *Standards of Practice for Clinical Pharmacists* (2014) and the American Association of Respiratory Care's *Respiratory Care Scope of Practice* (2018). These standards provide broad expectations for practice in all settings where healthcare is delivered and are translated into organization-specific standards such as policies, protocols, and procedures.

According to the IOM *Health Professions Education* summit report (2003), regardless of their discipline, all HCPs should have a core set of competencies that include the ability to use evidence-based practice, work in interdisciplinary teams, apply quality improvement methods, utilize informatics, and provide patient-centered care (see Figure 3.2). These competencies are achieved using consistent communication skills, obtaining knowledge and skills, and using clinical reasoning and reflection routinely in the practice setting.

The *Health Professions Education* report's core competencies support the use of interprofessional team collaboration in which a variety of diverse professionals share their observations and knowledge through communication and collaboration. Both EBP and research initiatives have become more interprofessional in nature, and interdisciplinary teams have been shown to enhance quality outcomes through the integration of professional perspectives, lower costs, and improve interactions among team members, thereby promoting patient safety and reducing medical errors (Aein et al., 2020; Bohnenkamp et al., 2014; IOM, 2003). Working in interprofessional teams allows all team members to contribute their expertise to achieve the best possible outcomes for patients and fosters role appreciation and job satisfaction between team members (Bohnenkamp et al., 2014). Practice change and improvement will also be more readily accepted within the organization and by all disciplines when it is based on evidence that has been evaluated through an interprofessional EBP process. An organization's ability to create opportunities for HCPs as part of an interprofessional team to develop EBP questions, evaluate evidence, promote critical thinking, make practice changes, and promote professional development is no longer optional.

Overlap of Core Competencies for Health Professionals

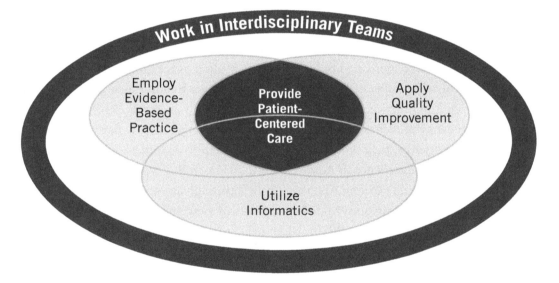

Figure 3.2 Relationship among core competencies for health professionals.
Copyright 2003 by the National Academy of Sciences. All rights reserved.

The use of an evidence-based approach in developing clinical practice standards and guidelines is also an expectation of regulatory agencies such as the Joint Commission (Joint Commission International, 2016) and for certifying bodies such as the American Nurses Credentialing Center [ANCC], which reviews organizations for Magnet Certification (ANCC, 2011). For example, healthcare organizations are standardizing practices based on evidence to reduce variations in care and practice to improve patient safety and quality while reducing healthcare costs (James, 2018; Warren et al., 2016).

Learning

According to Braungart et al. (2014), *learning* is "a relatively permanent change in mental processes, emotional functioning, skill, and/or behavior as a result of experience" (p. 64). Learning incorporates the active process of observing, interacting with phenomena, and engaging with others (Teaching Excellence in Adult Literacy, 2011). It builds on prior knowledge and often occurs in a complex social environment in which knowledge is built by engaged members. Learning requires the learner to be motivated to learn because it often uses significant mental energy and involves persistence. Learning allows the learner to adopt new knowledge by applying it in practice, resulting in behavior change (Lancaster, 2016). In addition to behavioral changes, learning can lead to changes in how participants think about themselves, their world, and others, referred to as *transformational learning* (Teaching Excellence in Adult Literacy, 2011). In this type of learning, critical reflection is used to examine issues or beliefs through assessing the evidence and arguments and being open to differing points of view and new information (Western Governors University, 2020). Ultimately, learning is what the learner hears and understands (Holmen, 2014).

A *learning culture* is a culture of inquiry that inspires staff to increase their knowledge, to develop new skills (Linders, 2014; McCormick, 2016), to support a growth mindset, and to believe that a person can acquire new skills and knowledge over time (Psychology Today, 2021). Staff with a growth mindset tend to actively seek out challenges and believe their true potential can be achieved through effort. Learning cultures also improve employee engagement, increase employee satisfaction, promote creativity, and encourage problem-solving (McCormick, 2016; Nabong, 2015). Both individual learning and a culture of learning are necessary to build practice expertise and maintain staff competency. Education is different from learning in that *education* imparts knowledge through teaching at a point in time, often in a formal setting. Education makes knowledge available.

According to Prabhat (2010), education is largely considered formal and shapes resources from the top down. Formalized education starts with an accredited institution that provides resources to meet that expressed goal. In contrast, learning begins with individuals and communities. The desire to learn, a natural desire, is considered informal learning and is based on the interests of individuals or groups who access resources in pursuit of that interest.

Ongoing learning is necessary to remain current with new knowledge, technologies, skills, and clinical competencies. Learning also serves to inform practice, which leads to changes in care standards that drive improvements in patient outcomes. Because the field of healthcare is becoming increasingly more complex and technical, no single individual can know everything about how best to provide safe and effective care, and no single degree can provide the knowledge needed to span an entire career. It is, therefore, an essential expectation that healthcare clinicians participate in lifelong learning and continued competency development (IOM, 2011).

"Education is what people do to you. Learning is what you do for yourself."

–Joi Ito

Lifelong learning is not only individual learning but also interprofessional, collaborative, and team-oriented learning. For example, joint learning experiences between nursing, medical, and pharmacy students facilitate a better understanding of roles and responsibilities, make communication more effective, aid in conflict resolution, and foster shared decision-making. They can also improve collaboration and the ability to work more effectively on interprofessional EBP teams. Interprofessional education and learning experiences foster collaboration, improve services, and prepare teams to solve problems using an EBP approach that exceeds the capacity of any single professional (Aein et al., 2020; IOM, 2011).

The JHEBP Model—Description

The JHEBP Model is an inquiry-based learning framework (Pedaste et al., 2015), in which individuals or interprofessional teams actively control their own learning to gain new knowledge and to update existing knowledge (Jong, 2006). This approach emphasizes the learner's role in the process, instead of a teacher telling learners what they need to know. Learners or teams are encouraged to explore, ask questions, and share ideas (Grade Power, 2018). The inquiry-learning process often starts with the investigation of a specific topic or problem to determine what currently is known and where there are gaps in knowledge. This phase may be followed by the development of an inquiry question or hypothesis leading to a plan to address the question through observation, the collection of evidence, experimentation, or data analysis (Jong, 2006; Pedaste et al., 2015). Based on the findings, conclusions are drawn and communicated. Future phases may include applying knowledge to new situations followed by evaluation. Reflection, which involves describing, critiquing, evaluating, and discussing, is an integral part of all phases of the inquiry-learning model. Reflection by learners leads to deeper learning and the ability to internalize complex knowledge (Kori et al., 2014). Examples of reflective questions might include:

1. What do we need to know about a particular problem?
2. How can we find the information that we need?
3. Are the resources used reliable?
4. What were the barriers in the process?
5. What could be done differently the next time to improve the process?

An inquiry-learning framework has its foundation in the work of earlier theorists such as Dewey and Piaget, whose learning philosophies were based on belief that experience provides the best process for acquiring knowledge (Barrow, 2006; Zaphir, 2019). Learners are encouraged to be self-directed based on personal experiences, and participate in group collaboration as well as in peer grading or review. A second learning philosophy—*connectivism*—evolving from the development and rapid growth of digital technology (Duke et al., 2013) includes concepts such as self-directed social learning, content sharing, and group collaboration. Technology allows learners to access a large array of concepts networked by information sets. The core skill then for the learner is to be able to identify connections between information sources and to maintain those connections to facilitate continual learning because data is constantly changing and updating (Duke et al., 2013).

Inquiry is the starting point for the JHEBP model (refer to Figure 3.1). An individual or a team, sparked by a genuine spirit of curiosity, seeks to clarify practice concerns by reflecting on such questions as whether current practices are based on the best evidence for a specific problem or a particular patient population, or perhaps considering whether there is a more efficient and cost-effective way of achieving a particular outcome. The PET (Practice Question, Evidence, and Translation) process shown in the EBP model provides a systematic approach for developing a practice question, finding the best evidence, and translating best evidence into practice. As the individual or team moves through the PET process, they are continually learning by gaining new knowledge, improving skills in collaboration, and gaining insights. These insights generate new EBP questions for future investigation at any time throughout the EBP process. The model also depicts that practice improvements are often clinical, learning, or operational in nature and are based on the translation of best evidence into practice. The ongoing cycle of inquiry, practice, and learning; identifying best evidence; and implementing practice improvements makes the JHEBP model a dynamic and interactive process for making practice changes that impact system, nurse, and patient outcomes. As depicted in the model, reflection by the team based on their discipline perspective and experiences serves to deepen learning through intentional discourse and articulation of important lessons learned throughout the entire EBP process (Di Stefano et al., 2014).

Critical Thinking, Clinical Reasoning, and Evidence-Based Practice

The ability of the EBP team to apply elements of critical thinking and clinical reasoning to the EBP process is vital to the success of any EBP project because it ensures that outcomes are based on sound evidence (Canada, 2016; Finn, 2011; Kim et al., 2018; Profetto-McGrath, 2005). *Critical thinking* is the process of questioning, analysis, synthesis, interpretation, inference, reasoning, intuition, application, and creativity (AACN, 2008). It is a means of imposing intellectual standards in the approach to any subject in a non-discipline-specific way (Victor-Chmil, 2013). *Clinical reasoning* employs critical thinking in the cognitive process that is used by healthcare professionals when examining a patient care concern (Victor-Chmil, 2013). Critical thinkers bring a variety of skills to the EBP team that help to effectively support the EBP process. They see problems from differing perspectives, use a variety of investigative approaches, and generate many ideas before developing a plan of action (Murawski, 2014). They see problems as challenges, rely on evidence to make judgments, are interested in what others have to say, think before acting, and engage in active listening.

When critical thinking skills are applied to the EBP process, a team is more apt to examine problems carefully, clarify assumptions and biases, and identify any missing information (Herr, 2007). The team uses critical thinking when determining the strength and quality of the evidence and the quantity and consistency of the evidence and then combines these findings to determine the best evidence recommendations, a process referred to as *synthesis*. Critical thinking fosters the use of logic to evaluate arguments, gather facts, weigh the evidence, and arrive at conclusions.

Based on this sound process, the EBP team uses clinical reasoning to think beyond traditional patient care routines and protocols and engage in critical analysis of current healthcare practices to determine the relevance of the evidence as it applies to a specific clinical situation (Profetto-McGrath, 2005; Victor-Chmil, 2013). For example, consider how clinical reasoning skills might be used by an EBP team looking at how hourly rounding impacts fall rates and patient satisfaction with nurse responsiveness. In developing the EBP question, the team employs clinical reasoning when questioning if they have a full understanding of the current practices on the nursing units impacted by the project and what additional information might be needed. The team may consider if they have gathered all available data that substantiates the problem (e.g., current fall rates, falls with injuries, and Health Consumer Assessment of Healthcare Providers and Systems [HCAHPS] scores). The team may also examine differences between different levels of care (e.g., critical, acute, or behavioral care). The team must also determine whether the recommendations for translation are a good fit for the clinical area and stakeholders, are feasible to implement in the identified areas, and are deemed acceptable within the organization.

Factors Influencing the JHEBP Model

The JHEBP Model is an open system with interrelated components. Because it is an open system, inquiry, learning, and practice are influenced by not only evidence but also factors external and internal to the organization. *External factors* can include accreditation bodies, legislation, quality measures, regulations, and standards. Accreditation bodies (e.g., The Joint Commission, Commission on Accreditation of Rehabilitation Facilities) require an organization to achieve and maintain high standards of practice and quality. Legislative and regulatory bodies (local, state, and federal) enact laws and regulations designed to protect the public and promote access to safe, quality healthcare services. Failure to adhere to these laws and regulations has adverse effects on an organization, most often financial. Examples of regulatory agencies are the Centers for Medicare & Medicaid Services, Food and Drug Administration, and state boards of nursing. State boards of nursing regulate nursing practice and enforce the Nurse Practice Act, which serves to protect the public. Quality measures (outcome and performance data) and professional standards serve as yardsticks for evaluating current practice and identifying areas for improvement or change. The American Nurses Credentialing Center, through its Magnet Recognition Program, developed criteria to assess the quality of nursing and nursing excellence in organizations. Additionally, many external stakeholders such as healthcare networks, special interest groups/organizations, vendors, patients and their families, the community, and third-party payors exert influence on healthcare organizations.

Internal factors can include organizational culture, values, and beliefs; practice environment (e.g., leadership, resource allocation, patient services, organizational mission and priorities, availability of technology, library support, time to conduct EBP activities); equipment and supplies; staffing; and organizational standards. Enacting EBP within an organization requires:

- A culture that believes EBP will lead to optimal patient outcomes
- A culture that supports interprofessional collaboration
- Strong and visible leadership support at all levels with the necessary resources (human, technological, and financial) to sustain the process

- Clear expectations that incorporate EBP into standards and job descriptions
- Availability of EBP mentors such as unit-based EBP champions, advanced practice clinicians and those with practice doctorates in nursing, pharmacy, and physical therapy, for example, and other organizational experts in the EBP process to serve as coaches and role models

Partnerships and interprofessional collaboration are crucial for the implementation of EBP initiatives that align with a healthcare organization's mission, goals, and strategic priorities (Moch et al., 2015). Mentors with knowledge of the patient population and the context of internal and external factors are essential for successful implementation and sustainability of EBP.

JHEBP PET Process: Practice Question, Evidence, and Translation

The JHEBP process occurs in three phases and can be simply described as Practice Question, Evidence, and Translation (PET) (see Figure 3.3). The 20-step process (see Appendix A) begins with the recruitment of an EBP team interested in examining a specific concern, followed by determining team leadership/responsibilities and meeting schedule. Next, clarify and describe the practice problem, issue, or concern. This step is critical because the problem statement drives the remaining steps in the process. Based on the problem statement, the EBP team develops a practice question; refines it; and searches for, appraises, and synthesizes the evidence. Through synthesis, the team decides whether the evidence supports a change in practice. If it does, evidence translation begins and the practice change is planned, implemented, and evaluated. The final step in translation is the dissemination of results to patients and their families, staff, hospital stakeholders, and, if appropriate, the local and national community.

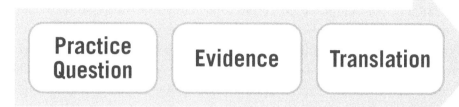

© The Johns Hopkins Health System/The Johns Hopkins University School of Nursing

Figure 3.3   JHEBP PET process: Practice Question, Evidence, and Translation.

Practice Question

The first phase of the process (Steps 1–7) includes forming a team and developing an answerable EBP question. An interprofessional team examines a practice concern, develops and refines an EBP question, and determines its scope. Refer to the PET Process Guide (see Appendix A) frequently throughout the process to direct the team's work and gauge progress. The tool identifies the following steps.

Step 1: Recruit Interprofessional Team

The first step in the EBP process is to form an interprofessional team to examine a specific practice concern. It is important to recruit members for which the practice concern holds relevance. When members are interested and invested in addressing a specific practice concern, they are generally more effective as a team. Frontline clinicians are key members because they have firsthand knowledge of the problem, its context, and its impact. Other relevant stakeholders may include team members such as clinical specialists (nursing or pharmacy), members of committees or ancillary departments, physicians, dieticians, pharmacists, patients, and families. These stakeholders may provide discipline-specific expertise or insights to create the most comprehensive view of the problem and, thus, the most relevant practice question. Keeping the group size to six to eight members makes it easier to schedule meetings and helps to maximize participation.

Step 2: Determine Responsibility for Project Leadership

Identifying a leader for the EBP project facilitates the process, accountabilities, and responsibilities and keeps the project moving forward. The ideal leader is knowledgeable about evidence-based practice and has experience and a proven track record in leading interprofessional teams. It is also helpful if this individual knows the structure and strategies for implementing change within the organization.

Step 3: Schedule Team Meetings

The leader takes initial responsibility to set up the first EBP team meeting and involves members in the following activities:

- Reserving a room with adequate space conducive to group work and discussion
- Asking team members to bring their calendars so that subsequent meetings can be scheduled
- Ensuring that a team member is assigned to record discussion points and group decisions
- Establishing a project plan and timeline for the project
- Keeping track of important items (e.g., copies of the EBP tools, literature searches, materials, and resources)
- Providing a place to keep project files

Step 4: Clarify and Describe the Problem

To define a problem accurately, the EBP team invests time to identify the gap between the current practice and the desired practice—in other words, between what the team sees and experiences and what they want to see and experience. This is accomplished by stating the problem in different ways and soliciting feedback from nonmembers to see whether there is agreement on the problem statement. Teams should gather information, both narrative and numerical, to identify why the current practice is a problem. To do this, team members might observe the practice and listen to how actual users describe the problem in comparison to anticipated practice changes. The time devoted to probing issues and challenging assumptions about the problem, looking at it from multiple angles and obtaining feedback from as many sources as possible, is always time well spent. Incorrectly identifying the problem results in wasted effort searching and appraising evidence that, in the end, does not provide the insight that allows the team to achieve the desired outcomes.

Step 5: Develop and Refine the EBP Question

With a problem statement clearly stated, the EBP team develops and refines the clinical, learning, or operational EBP question (see Appendix B). Keeping the EBP question narrowly focused makes the search for evidence specific and manageable. For example, the question, "What is the best way to stop the transmission of methicillin-resistant Staphylococcus aureus (MRSA)?" is extremely broad and could encompass many interventions and all practice settings. This type of question, known as a background question, is often used when the team knows little about the area of concern or is interested in identifying best practices. In contrast, a more focused question is, "What works best in the critical-care setting to prevent the spread of MRSA—hand washing with soap and water or the use of alcohol-based hand sanitizers?" This type of question, known as a foreground question, is generally used by more experienced teams with specialized knowledge to compare interventions or make decisions. In general, foreground questions are narrow and allow the search for evidence to be more precise and focused.

The PET process uses the PICO mnemonic (Sackett et al., 2000) to describe the four elements of a focused question: (a) **patient**, population, or problem, (b) **intervention**, (c) **comparison** with other interventions, and (d) measurable **outcomes** (see Table 3.1).

Table 3.1   Application of PICO Elements

Patient, population, or problem
Team members determine the specific patient, population, or problem related to the patient/population for the topic of concern. Examples include age, sex, ethnicity, condition, disease, and setting.

Intervention
Team members identify the specific intervention or approach to be examined. Examples include treatments, protocols, education, self-care, and best practices.

Comparison with other interventions, if applicable
Team members identify what they are comparing the intervention to—for example, current practice or another intervention.

Outcomes
Team members identify expected outcomes based on the implementation of a change in practice/intervention. The outcomes (measures of structure, process, outcomes) determine the effectiveness of a change or improvement.

Using this format, the Question Development Tool (see Appendix B) guides the team to define the practice problem, examine current practice, identify how and why the problem was selected, limit the scope of the problem, and narrow the EBP question. The tool also helps the team to determine a search strategy, sources of evidence that will be searched, inclusion and exclusion criteria, and possible search terms. EBP teams can go back and further refine the EBP question as they gain more information during the evidence search and review.

Step 6: Determine the Need for an EBP Project

Prior to proceeding with the EBP process, the team should conduct a preliminary scan of the literature to determine the presence or absence of research evidence related to the identified problem. If there is a high-quality, current (within five years) systematic review, such as a Cochrane Review, the EBP team determines whether the review is sufficient to address the EBP problem or whether an EBP project is still warranted. If the preliminary scan indicates a lack of research related to the problem, consideration should be given to whether a quality improvement project or conducting a research study would be the most effective way of addressing the problem. Other options, in the absence of research evidence, would include staying with current organizational practice or investigating/confirming the community standard. Only when the preliminary scan of the literature indicates that it is likely that sufficient research evidence is available should the team move forward with the EBP project (see the decision tree in Appendix A).

Step 7: Identify Stakeholders

It is important for the EBP team to identify early the appropriate individuals and stakeholders who should be involved in and kept informed during the EBP project. A *stakeholder* is a person, group, or department in an organization that has an interest in, or a concern about, the topic or project under consideration (Agency for Healthcare Research and Quality, 2011). Stakeholders may include a variety of clinical and nonclinical staff, departmental and organizational leaders, patients and families, regulators, insurers, or policymakers. Keeping key stakeholders informed is instrumental to successful change. The team also considers whether the EBP question is specific to a unit, service, or department or involves multiple departments. If it is the latter, representatives from all areas involved need to be recruited for the EBP team. The team regularly communicates with key leaders in the affected departments on the team's progress. If the problem affects multiple disciplines (e.g., nursing, medicine, pharmacy, respiratory therapy), these disciplines need to be a part of the team. The Stakeholder Analysis Tool in Appendix C is used to guide stakeholder identification.

Evidence

The second phase (Steps 8–12) of the PET process addresses the search for, appraisal of, and synthesis of the best available evidence. Based on these results, the team makes best evidence recommendations regarding practice changes.

Step 8: Conduct Internal and External Search for Evidence

Team members determine the type of evidence to search for (see Chapter 5), who is to conduct the search, and who will bring items to the committee for review. Enlisting the assistance of a health information specialist (librarian) is highly recommended. Such assistance saves time and ensures a comprehensive and relevant search. In addition to library resources, other sources of evidence include:

- Clinical practice guidelines
- Community standards
- Opinions of internal and external experts
- Organizational financial data
- Position statements from professional organizations
- Patient and staff surveys and satisfaction data
- Quality improvement data
- Regulatory, safety, or risk-management data

Step 9: Appraise the Level and Quality of Each Piece of Evidence

In this step, the team appraises the type of evidence (research and nonresearch) for level and quality. The Research Evidence Appraisal Tool (see Appendix E) and the Nonresearch Evidence Appraisal Tool (see Appendix F) assist the team in this activity. Each tool includes a set of questions to determine the level and quality of each piece of evidence. The JHEBP Model uses a five-level hierarchy to determine the level of the evidence, with Level I evidence as the highest and Level V as the lowest (see Appendix D). Based on the questions provided on the tools, the quality of each piece of evidence is rated as high, good, or low. Evidence with a quality rating of low is discarded and is not used in the process.

Step 10: Summarize the Individual Evidence

The Individual Evidence Summary Tool (see Appendix G) tracks the team's appraisal and summarization of each piece of evidence (including the author, date, evidence type, population, sample size, setting, intervention, study findings, measures used, limitations, and evidence level and quality). Chapters 6 and 7 provide a detailed discussion of evidence appraisal.

Step 11: Synthesize Findings

The EBP team applies critical thinking skills to deliberate and thoughtfully evaluate the body of evidence and come to agreement on the strength, quantity, and findings of the overall body of evidence. The overall quality for each level, number of evidence sources, and synthesized findings for each level are then recorded on the Synthesis and Recommendations Tool (see Appendix H).

Step 12: Develop Best Evidence Recommendations

To develop best evidence recommendations, the team employs the evidence synthesis results identified in Step 11 and the characteristics of the evidence as listed below. The team determines the evidence characteristics by obtaining agreement on which of the following statements best describes the overall body of the evidence:

- **Strong & compelling evidence, consistent results:** Recommendations are reliable; evaluate for organizational translation.
- **Good evidence & consistent results:** Recommendations may be reliable; evaluate for risk and organizational translation.
- **Good evidence but conflicting results:** Unable to establish best practice based on current evidence; evaluate risk, consider further investigation for new evidence, develop a research study, or discontinue the project.
- **Little or no evidence:** Unable to establish best practice based on current evidence; consider further investigation for new evidence, develop a research study, or discontinue the project.

Adapted from Poe and White (2010)

Based on the evidence synthesis and the evidence characteristics, the team next determines whether to make best evidence recommendations or whether additional investigation is needed. Best evidence recommendations are made based on strength, quantity, and consistency of the evidence and should not be made when little to no evidence exists. If the team decides to move forward with best evidence recommendations, the recommendations should be written as distinct statements that answer the EBP question. They are then recorded on the Synthesis and Recommendations Tool (see Appendix H). It is highly recommended that the EBP team pilot practice or improvement recommendations/changes in several representative areas/settings to determine possible unanticipated effects or barriers.

Translation

In the third phase (Steps 13–20) of the PET process, the EBP team determines the feasibility, fit, and acceptability of the best evidence recommendations within the target setting. When considering feasibility, the team determines the extent to which a change (system process improvement, innovation, or practice change) can be successfully implemented within a given organization or practice setting. Determination of fit includes the team's perceived relevance or compatibility of the change with the user's workflow for the given practice setting, provider, or consumer; and/or perceived relevance of the change to address a particular issue or problem. Lastly, acceptability is the team's perception regarding the extent to which stakeholders and organizational leadership perceives a change to be agreeable, palatable, and satisfactory for the organization. If the assessment for feasibility, fit, and acceptability is positive, the team proceeds with creating an action plan, secures support and resources, implements and evaluates the change, and communicates the results to appropriate individuals both internal and external to the organization.

Step 13: Identify Practice Setting–Specific Recommendations

The team communicates and obtains feedback from appropriate organizational leaders, bedside clinicians, and all other stakeholders affected by the practice recommendations to determine whether the change is feasible, is a good fit, and is acceptable given the specific practice setting and organization. They also consider the resources available and the organization's readiness for change (Poe & White, 2010). Even with strong, compelling evidence, EBP teams may find it difficult to implement practice changes in some cases. For example, an EBP team examined the best strategy for ensuring appropriate enteral tube placement after initial tube insertion. The evidence indicated that X-ray was the only 100% accurate method for identifying tube location. The EBP team recommended that a post-insertion X-ray be added to the enteral tube protocol. Despite their presenting the evidence to clinical leadership and other organizational stakeholders, the team's recommendation was not accepted within the organization. Concerns were raised by organizational leadership about the additional costs and adverse effects that may be incurred by patients (acceptability). Other concerns related to delays in workflow (fit) and the availability of staff to perform the additional X-rays (feasibility). Risk management data showed a lack of documented incidents related to inappropriate enteral tube placement. As a result, after weighing the risks and benefits, the organization decided that making this change was not a good fit at that time. The feasibility-fit-acceptability section of the Translation and Action Planning Tool (see Appendix I) provides statements to consider when determining the likelihood of being successful in these areas.

Step 14: Create Action Plan

In this step, the team develops a plan to implement the practice change(s). The plan may include, but is not limited to:

1. Development of (or change to) a standard (policy, protocol, guideline, or procedure), a critical pathway, or a system or process related to the EBP question.

2. Development of a detailed timeline assigning team members to the tasks needed to implement the change (including the evaluation process and reporting of results).

3. Solicitation of feedback from organizational leaders, bedside clinicians, and other stakeholders.

Essentially, the team must consider the who, what, when, where, how, and why when developing an action plan for the proposed change. The Action Planning section of the Translation and Action Planning Tool (see Appendix I) provides a guide for the EBP team to develop the action plan.

Step 15: Secure Support and Resources to Implement Action Plan

The team carefully and comprehensively considers the human, material, or financial resources needed to implement the action plan. Obtaining support and working closely with departmental and organizational leaders ensures successful implementation of the EBP action plan.

Step 16: Implement Action Plan

When the team implements the action plan, they need to make certain that all affected staff and stakeholders receive verbal and written communication as well as education about the practice change, implementation plan, and evaluation process. EBP team members need to be available to answer any questions and troubleshoot problems that may arise during implementation.

Step 17: If Change Is Implemented, Evaluate Outcomes to Determine Whether Improvements Have Been Made

Using the Outcomes Measurement Plan section of the Translation and Action Planning Tool (see Appendix I), the team evaluates the success of the change for both the pilot and broader adoption. Although the team desires positive outcomes, unexpected outcomes often provide opportunities for learning, and the team should examine why these occurred. This examination may indicate the need to alter the practice change or the implementation process, followed by re-evaluation.

One way to evaluate outcomes particularly for uncomplicated, small tests of change is through the quality improvement process. The Plan-Do-Study-Act (PDSA) quality improvement cycle is a tested way to determine whether a practice change has met desired outcomes/improvements (Institute for Healthcare

Improvement, 2020). When using the PDSA cycle, the team begins by planning the change, implementing it, observing the results, and then acting on what is learned. The process can help teams to determine whether the change brought about improvement; how much improvement can be expected; whether the change will work in the actual environment of interest; costs, social impact, and side effects of the change; and ways to minimize resistance to the change.

Step 18: Report Results to Stakeholders

In this step, the team reports the results to appropriate organizational leaders, frontline clinicians, and all other stakeholders. Sharing and disseminating the results, both favorable and unfavorable, may generate additional practice or research questions. Valuable feedback obtained from stakeholders can overcome barriers to implementation or help develop strategies to improve unfavorable results. The Stakeholder Analysis and Communication Tool (Appendix C) guides the EBP team in identifying the audience(s), key message points, and methods to communicate the team's findings, recommendations, and practice changes.

Step 19: Identify Next Steps

EBP team members review the process and findings and consider whether any lessons have emerged that should be shared or whether additional steps need to be taken. These lessons or steps may include a new question that has emerged from the process, the need to do more research on the topic, additional training that may be required, suggestions for new tools, the writing of an article on the process or outcome, or the preparation of an oral or poster presentation at a professional conference. The team may identify other problems that have no evidence base and, therefore, require the development of a research protocol. For example, when the recommendation to perform a chest X-ray to validate initial enteral tube placement was not accepted (see the example discussed in Step 13), the EBP team decided to design a research study to look at the use of colorimetric carbon dioxide detectors to determine tube location.

Step 20: Disseminate Findings

This final step of the translation process is one that is often overlooked and requires strong organizational support. The results of the EBP project need to be, at a minimum, communicated to the organization. Depending on the scope of the EBP question and the outcome, consideration should be given to communicating findings external to the organization in appropriate professional journals or through presentations at professional conferences. Refer to the Stakeholder Analysis and Communication Tool (Appendix C) and the Template for Publishing an Evidence-Based Practice Project (see Appendix J).

Summary

This chapter introduced the revised JHEBP Model (2020) and the steps of the PET process, designed as an intentional and systematic approach to EBP that requires support and commitment at the individual, team, and organizational levels. HCPs with varied experience and educational preparation have successfully used this process with coaching, mentorship, and organizational support (Dearholt & Dang, 2012).

References

Aein, F., Hosseini, R., Naseh, L., Safdari, F., & Banaian, S. (2020). The effect of problem-solving-based interprofessional learning on critical thinking and satisfaction with learning of nursing and midwifery students. *Journal of Education and Health Promotion*, 9(109). https://doi.org/10.4103/jehp.jehp_640_19

Agency for Healthcare Research and Quality. (2011). *Engaging stakeholders to identify and prioritize future research needs*. https://www.ncbi.nlm.nih.gov/books/NBK62565/pdf/Bookshelf_NBK62565.pdf

American Association of Colleges of Nursing. (2008). *The essentials of baccalaureate education for professional nursing practice*. http://www.aacnnursing.org/portals/42/publications/baccessentials08.pdf

American Association of Colleges of Nursing. (2020). *Nursing fact sheet*. https://www.aacnnursing.org/News-Information/Fact-Sheets/Nursing-Fact-Sheet

American Association of Respiratory Care. (2018). *Respiratory care scope of practice*. https://www.aarc.org/wp-content/uploads/2017/03/statement-of-scope-of-practice.pdf

American College of Clinical Pharmacy. (2014). *Standards of Practice for Clinical Pharmacists*. Pharmacotherapy, Aug;34(8):794-7. doi:10.1002/phar.1438. PMID: 25112523

American Nurses Association. (2010). *Nursing: Scope and standards of practice*. American Nurses Association.

American Nurses Association. (2015). *Nursing: Scope and standards of practice* (3rd ed.). American Nurses Association.

American Nurses Credentialing Center. (2011). *Announcing the model for ANCC's Magnet recognition program*. http://www.nursecredentialing.org/Magnet/ProgramOverview/New-Magnet-Model.aspx

Barrow, L. H. (2006). A brief history of inquiry: From Dewey to standards. *Journal of Science Teacher Education*, 17(3), 265–278. https://www.jstor.org/stable/43156392

Bohnenkamp, S., Pelton, N., Rishel, C. J., & Kurtin, S. (2014). Implementing evidence-based practice using an interprofessional team approach. *Oncology Nursing Forum*, 41(4), 434–437. https://doi.org/10.1188/14.ONF.434-437

Braungart, M., Braungart, R. G., & Gramet, P. R. (2014). Applying learning theories to healthcare practice. In S. B. Bastable (Ed.), *Nurse as educator, principles of teaching and learning for nursing practice* (pp. 64–110), Jones & Bartlett Learning.

Canada, A. N. (2016). Probing the relationship between evidence-based practice implementation models and critical thinking in applied nursing practice. *The Journal of Continuing Education in Nursing*, 47(4), 161–168. https://doi.org/10.3928/00220124-20160322-05

Dearholt, S. L., & Dang, D. (2012). *Johns Hopkins nursing evidence-based practice: Model and guidelines* (2nd ed.). Sigma Theta Tau International.

Di Stefano, G., Gino, F., Pisano, G., & Staats, B. (2014). Learning by thinking: How reflection improves performance. *Harvard Business School, Working Knowledge*. https://hbswk.hbs.edu/item/learning-by-thinking-how-reflection-improves-performance

Duke, B., Harper, G., & Johnston, M. (2013). Connectivism as a digital age learning theory. *The International HETL Review, Special Issue*. https://www.hetl.org/wp-content/uploads/2013/09/HETLReview2013 SpecialIssueArticle1.pdf

Finn, P. (2011). Critical thinking: Knowledge and skills for evidence-based practice. *Language, Speech, and Hearing Services in Schools*, 42, 69–72.

Grade Power. (2018, April 3). What is inquiry-based learning (and how is it effective)? *Grade Power Learning*. https://gradepowerlearning.com/what-is-inquiry-based-learning/

Herr, N. (2007). Critical thinking. *Internet Resources to Accompany the Sourcebook for Teaching Science*. https://www.csun.edu/science/ref/reasoning/critical_thinking/index.html

Holmen, M. (2014, August 6). Education vs learning—What exactly is the difference? *EdTechReview*. http://edtechreview.in/trends-insights/insights/1417-education-vs-learning-what-exactly-is-the-difference?utm_content=buffer4e5b8&utm_medium=social&utm_source=twitter.com&utm_campaign=buffer#.U-NdPce3yG4.twitter

Institute for Healthcare Improvement. (2020). *Science of improvement: Testing changes*. http://www.ihi.org/resources/Pages/HowtoImprove/ScienceofImprovementTestingChanges.aspx

Institute of Medicine. (2003). *Health professions education: A bridge to quality*. National Academies Press.

Institute of Medicine. (2009). *Roundtable on evidence-based medicine*. National Academies Press. https://www.ncbi.nlm.nih.gov/books/NBK52847

Institute of Medicine. (2011). *The future of nursing: Leading change, advancing health*. The National Academics Press.

James, T. (2018). The science of health care improvement: Overcoming unintended variation. *Harvard Medical School Lean Forward*. https://leanforward.hms.harvard.edu/2018/11/29/the-science-of-health-care-improvement-overcoming-unintended-variation/

Joint Commission International (2016). *Clinical practice guidelines: Closing the gap between theory and practice*. https://www.elsevier.com/__data/assets/pdf_file/0007/190177/JCI-Whitepaper_cpgs-closing-the-gap.pdf

Jong, T. (2006). Technological advances in inquiry learning. *Science, 312*(5773), 532–533.

Kim, S. S., Kim, E. J., Lim, J. Y., Kim, G. M., & Baek, H. C. (2018). Korean nursing students' acquisition of evidence-based practice and critical thinking skills. *Journal of Nursing Education, 57*(1), 21–27. https://doi.org/10.3928/01484834-20180102-05

Kori, K., Maeots, M., & Pedaste, M. (2014). Guided reflection to support quality of reflection and inquiry in web-based learning. *Procedia: Social and Behavioral Sciences, 112*, 242–251. https://www.sciencedirect.com/science/article/pii/S1877042814011781

Lancaster, J. (2016). Changing health behavior using health education with individuals, families, and groups. In M. Stanhope & J. Lancaster (Eds.), *Public health nursing* (pp. 355–376). Elsevier Mosby.

Linders, B. (2014, July 24). Nurturing a culture for continuous learning. *InfoQ*. https://www.infoq.com/news/2014/07/nurture-culture-learning

McCormick, H. (2016). *Seven steps to creating a lasting learning culture*. University of North Carolina. http://execdev.kenan-flagler.unc.edu/hubfs/White%20Papers/unc-white-paper-7-steps-to-creating-a-lasting-learning-culture.pdf

Melnyk, B. M., Fineout-Overholt, E., Stillwell, S. B., & Williamson, K. M. (2009). Igniting a spirit of inquiry: An essential foundation for evidence-based practice. *American Journal of Nursing, 109*(11), 49–52.

Migliore, L., Chouinard, H., & Woodlee, R. (2020). Clinical research and practice collaborative: An evidence-based nursing clinical inquiry expansion. *Military Medicine, 185*(2), 35–42. https://doi.org/10.1093/milmed/usz447

Moch, S. D., Quinn-Lee, L., Gallegos, C., & Sortedahl, C. K. (2015). Navigating evidence-based practice projects: The faculty role. *Nursing Education Perspectives, 36*(2), 128–130. https://doi.org/10.5480/12-1014.1

Murawski, L. M. (2014). Critical thinking in the classroom . . . and beyond. *Journal of Learning in Higher Education, 10*(1), 25–30.

Nabong, T. (2015, April 7). Creating a learning culture for the improvement of your organization. *Training Industry*. https://www.trainingindustry.com/workforce-development/articles/creating-a-learning-culture-for-the-improvement-of-your-organization.aspx

National League for Nursing. (2014). *Practical/vocational nursing program outcome: Spirit of inquiry*. http://www.nln.org/docs/default-source/default-document-library/spirit-of-inquiry-final.pdf?sfvrsn=0

Pedaste, M., Maeots, M., Siiman, L. A., Jong, T., Van Riesen, S., Kamp, E. T., Manoli, C. C., Zacharia, Z. C., & Tsourlidaki, E. (2015). Phases of inquiry-based learning: Definitions and the inquiry cycle. *Educational Research Review*, *14*(2015), 47–61. https://doi.org/10.1016/j.edurev.2015.02.003

Poe, S. S., & White, K. M. (2010). *Johns Hopkins Nursing Evidence-Based Practice: Implementation and translation*. Sigma Theta Tau International.

Prabhat, S. (2010, January 26). Difference between education and learning. *Difference Between*. http://www.differencebetween.net/miscellaneous/difference-between-education-and-learning

Profetto-McGrath, J. (2005). Critical thinking and evidence-based practice. *Journal of Professional Nursing*, *21*(6), 364–371. https://doi.org/10.1016/j.profnurs.2005.10.002

Psychology Today. (2021). Growth mindset: What is a growth mindset? https://www.psychologytoday.com/us/basics/growth-mindset

Sackett, D. L., Straus, S. E., Richardson, W. S., Rosenberg, W., & Haynes, R. B. (2000). *Evidence-based medicine: How to practice and teach EBM*. Churchill.

Saunders, H., Gallagher-Ford, L., Kvist, T., & Vehvilainen-Julkunen, K. (2019). Practicing HCPs' evidence-based practice competencies: An overview of systematic reviews. *Worldviews on Evidence-Based Nursing*, *16*(3), 176–185. https://doi.org/10.1111/wvn.12363

Teaching Excellence in Adult Literacy. (2011). *Adult learning theories*. https://lincs.ed.gov/sites/default/files/11_%20TEAL_Adult_Learning_Theory.pdf

Victor-Chmil, J. (2013). Critical thinking versus clinical reasoning versus clinical judgment: Differential diagnosis. *Nurse Educator*, *38*(1), 34–36. https://doi.org/10.1097/NNE.0b013e318276dfbe

Warren, J. I., McLaughlin, M., Bardsley, J., Eich, J., Esche, C. A., Kropkowski, L., & Risch, S. (2016). The strengths and challenges of implementing EBP in healthcare systems. *Worldviews on Evidence-Based Nursing*, *13*(1), 15–24.

Western Governors University. (2020, July 17). What is the transformative learning theory? *WGU Blog*. https://www.wgu.edu/blog/what-transformative-learning-theory2007.html

Wilson, M., Sleutel, M., Newcomb, P., Behan, D., Walsh, J., Wells, J. N., & Baldwin, K. M. (2015). Empowering nurses with evidence-based practice environments: Surveying Magnet, Pathway to Excellence, and non-Magnet facilities in one healthcare system. *Worldviews on Evidence-Based Nursing*, *12*(1), 12–21. https://doi.org/10.1111/wvn.12077

Zaphir, L. (2019, December 12). Knowledge is a process of discovery: How constructivism changed education. *The Conversation*. https://theconversation.com/knowledge-is-a-process-of-discovery-how-constructivism-changed-education-126585

Practice Question, Evidence, Translation (PET)

4 The Practice Question Phase. 73

5 Searching for Evidence. 99

6 Evidence Appraisal: Research 129

7 Evidence Appraisal: Nonresearch. 163

8 Translation 189

9 Dissemination 207

The Practice Question Phase

Practice questions frequently arise from day-to-day problems encountered by clinicians, leaders, administrators, and educators. Answers to these questions in the form of evidence are available in print or by way of electronic media or evidence summaries such as systematic reviews, integrative reviews, literature reviews, and guidelines. The objectives of this chapter are to help you:

- Identify the steps in forming an EBP team
- Define practice problems appropriate for an EBP approach
- Explore considerations for determining the need for an EBP project
- Use the PICO framework to create an answerable EBP question
- Identify appropriate stakeholders to ensure the success of the EBP project

The practice question phase of the PET process (Practice Question, Evidence, Translation) includes seven operational steps, shown in Box 4.1. The first step is to assemble an interprofessional team to examine a specific practice concern or problem. Team members work together to select a project leader, assign team responsibilities, and develop the meeting schedule. Then they define and develop a comprehensive understanding of the problem, determine the need for the EBP project, and identify stakeholders. The Johns Hopkins Evidence-Based Practice (JHNEBP) Question Development Tool (see Appendix B) facilitates this phase.

> **Box 4.1 Steps in Practice Question Phase—the P in PET Process**
>
> Step 1: Recruit interprofessional team.
> Step 2: Determine responsibility for project leadership.
> Step 3: Schedule team meetings.
> Step 4: Clarify and describe the problem.
> Step 5: Develop and refine the EBP question.
> Step 6: Determine the need for an EBP project.
> Step 7: Identify stakeholders.

The Interprofessional EBP Team

In 2003, the Institute of Medicine (IOM) commissioned a Consensus Study to identify competencies for health professions to deal with the increasing complexity of care, keep pace with the demands of new technology, respond to the demands of payors, and deliver care across settings. To this end, they proposed five "core competencies that all health clinicians should possess, regardless of their discipline, to meet the needs of the 21st-century health care system" (pp. 45–46):

- Provide patient-centered care
- Work in interdisciplinary teams
- Employ evidence-based practice
- Apply quality improvement
- Utilize informatics

Since then, the best evidence indicates that interprofessional teams do produce higher-quality patient care with better outcomes than healthcare professionals who provide care in silos (IOM, 2013).

In 2015, the Robert Wood Johnson Foundation conducted a study to identify best practices in real-world interprofessional team collaboration as (p. 1):

- Effective interprofessional collaboration promotes the active participation of each discipline in patient care, where all disciplines are working together, fully engaging patients and those who support them, and leadership on the team adapts based on patient needs.

- Effective interprofessional collaboration enhances patient- and family-centered goals and values, provides a mechanism for continuous communication among caregivers, and optimizes participation in clinical decision-making within and across the disciplines. It fosters respect for the disciplinary contributions of all professionals.

These findings have implications for building interprofessional evidence-based practice teams with members from different disciplines who contribute their varied and specialized knowledge, skills, and methods. Throughout the project, team members integrate their observations, bodies of expertise, and decision-making to coordinate, collaborate, and translate evidence into practice.

Building the EBP Team

The range of disciplines of EBP team members depends on the focus and scope of the problem. Anticipating whose practice may be affected is a good starting point for identifying colleagues as members or as stakeholders. The number of members should be small enough to promote efficiency and large enough to provide content expertise—ideally between six and eight people.

The next step is to determine the behaviors, skills, and expertise needed within the interprofessional EBP team. The team uses this information to select and invite colleagues with the requisite expertise to ensure the membership is inclusive. For example, if the question relates to best practices in the management of nausea for the patient undergoing chemotherapy, the team may consist of nurses, pharmacists, and oncologists.

Building a team with deliberate attention to the attributes of team members will ensure comprehensive perspectives, tight collaborations, and robust recommendations.

> **Box 4.2 Five Categories of Adopters**
>
> Rogers's Theory of Diffusion of Innovation (Rogers, 2003) describes five categories of adopters who can assist or delay adoption of improvements or changes in practice. Identifying those individuals who are considered late majority or laggards and inviting them to join the EBP team allows those individuals to be a part of the process and learn about the project in stages. This strategy may influence the late majority and laggard members to adopt evidence recommendations more readily.
>
> Categories of adopters are as follows:
>
> - **Innovators:** People in this category tend to be risk-takers motivated by being a change agent. This is about 2.5% of all people.
> - **Early adopters:** These people tend to be adventurous, trendsetters, opinion leaders, and role models respected by their peers. They compose 13.5% of the population.
> - **Early majority:** People in this category are also opinion leaders, but they tend to be more pragmatic and seek reliability to avoid risk. The early majority represents 34% of the population.
> - **Late majority:** These people tend to be more cautious or skeptical and can be easily influenced by laggards. This is about 34% of all people.
> - **Laggards:** People in this category tend to be suspicious, often favoring the status quo rather than change. They compose 16% of the population.

Figure 4.1 represents an example from a Pediatric Intensive Care Unit (PICU) implementing an EBP project providing telemedicine support to novice bedside nurses. Given the innovative nature of the EBP question, the initial EBP team recognized the need to thoughtfully recruit additional team members with consideration to their informal adopter role based on Rogers's theory (see Box 4.2). Informal adopter roles were assigned based on previous experience working with those individuals on other projects and day-to-day work.

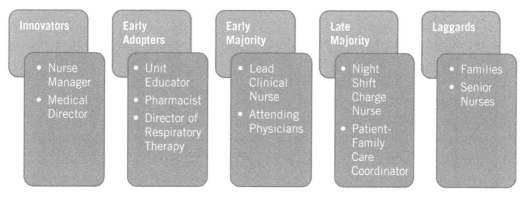

Figure 4.1 Example of PICU staff placement on the adopter curve.

Another consideration is to include both formal and informal leaders as EBP team members. Formal leaders differ from informal leaders in that formal leaders' roles and power are well defined by their position title in the organization. In contrast, informal leaders' influence is not a result of their position or title. Rather, they are clinical experts and unit historians that staff look to for answers and information. Formal leaders may be valuable during the EBP process by securing resources or funding and eliminating barriers.

Informal leaders in organizations are often identified as opinion leaders and change champions. Table 4.1 outlines characteristics of both opinion leaders and change champions. An effective EBP team should include both formal and informal leaders.

Table 4.1 Characteristics of Informal Leaders

Opinion Leaders	Change Champions
Part of local peer group	Within the local group settings (clinic, care unit)
Wide sphere of influence	Expert clinicians with positive relations with other professionals
Trusted to judge fit between innovation and unit norms	Encourage peers to adopt innovations, are persistent and passionate about innovation
Use of innovation influences peers and alters group norms	

In addition to understanding the roles of team members, it is equally important to understand the dynamics of an effective team. In 2008, Google collaborated with scientists from MIT on Project Aristotle (re:Work, 2020) to define the most important qualities of a productive team. The top five team dynamics include (re:Work, 2020):

- **Psychological safety:** Creating an environment that supports risk-taking and allows team members to feel safe expressing their vulnerability
- **Dependability:** Team members achieve goals and strive for excellence
- **Structure and clarity:** Team members have a clear expectation of their roles and responsibilities
- **Meaning:** Team members find importance in the project or their role on the team
- **Impact:** Seeing that the project is valuable and makes a difference

Role of the EBP Team

Team members' responsibilities are to contribute and support the team by attending meetings, reviewing and presenting evidence, participating in evidence synthesis, and generating practice recommendations through consensus building. Teams that have little to no experience with conducting an EBP project can benefit by inviting an experienced mentor to help them complete the process the first time.

The first decision that the newly formed team makes is to identify which member will serve as the team leader. The leader's responsibilities include coordinating meetings, guiding the project steps, articulating the team's recommendations, and influencing implementation through targeted communication. The leader guides team decision-making to establish a regular meeting schedule so that members can adjust their schedules ahead of time, to select a time and venue away from the demands of the clinical area, and to set a realistic timeline to complete the project. Team members who work multiple shifts, various days, and in different roles often require a long lead time to create space for this project work. Occasionally, teams can use a portion of regularly scheduled meetings (e.g., quality improvement, policy and procedure review, or other leadership meetings) for the EBP project. To be respectful of team members' time and competing priorities, the leader ensures the purpose and outcome of each meeting are clear and value-added. Effective leaders use email or other electronic channels to share information and ensure meeting accomplishments are documented and accessible for reference throughout the project to all team members. Leading productive team meetings is both an art and a skill even for experienced team leaders. The core practices of a good leader are:

1. Stay neutral; take no stake in the outcome of discussions.

2. Ask questions to test assumptions or to get to the root cause.

3. Actively listen; listen to understand—do not judge.

4. Continuously paraphrase; repeat what team members say to clarify.

5. Summarize discussions; this ensures the rest of the team has heard all the ideas, improves accuracy, and allows closure.

6. Record ideas with accurate notes that summarize discussions.

7. Synthesize ideas; allow team members' ideas to build upon one another's.

8. Keep on track; when discussions lose focus, the facilitator guides the team back.

9. Test assumptions; make sure these are surfaced and validated.
10. Manage the climate; create a collaborative team through structure (i.e., team norms/behaviors).

Some teams schedule a preliminary meeting to refine the practice problem and question and then one or two eight-hour days to review the evidence and make recommendations. Others have approached scheduling challenges by setting aside four-hour blocks of time monthly or five two-hour meetings every other week. Scheduling meetings weekly or every two weeks keeps the team moving forward. Delays between group meetings diminish the team's momentum.

The EBP team leader designates responsibility for the subsequent steps in the EBP process. Action items may include inviting new members to the team, reporting to internal committees, or providing information to organizational leaders about the EBP project.

Another useful strategy for the leader to sustain team momentum is the use of action plans, work breakdown structures, or Gantt charts to guide and structure the project work. The PET Process Guide (Appendix A) provides a useful tracking tool for each step of the EBP process. Without this planning and coordination, precious time and resources can be wasted and lead to an unsuccessful EBP project.

Clarifying and Describing the Practice Problem

Once assembled, the interprofessional team members begin by defining the practice problem. Describing the problem precisely and succinctly is essential because all subsequent actions and decisions build on the clarity and accuracy of the problem statement. The wrong problem will result in the wrong solution. The process often begins by seeking answers to practice concerns such as:

- Is there evidence that this intervention works?
- How does this practice help the patient?
- Why are we doing this practice, and should we be doing it this way?

- Is there a way to improve this practice so that it is more efficient or more cost-effective?
- How can we improve the quality, safety, and cost of our practice?

EBP questions can emerge from multiple sources. Titler et al., in two classic publications (1994, 2001), identified sources of problems to come from triggers that are problem-focused or knowledge-focused. *Problem-focused triggers* are identified by staff during routine monitoring of quality, risk, financial, or benchmarking data or adverse events. *Knowledge-focused triggers* are identified by reading published reports or learning new information at conferences or professional meetings (see Table 4.2).

Table 4.2 Sources of Evidence-Based Practice Problems

Trigger	Sources of Evidence-Based Practice Problems
Problem-focused	Financial concerns
	Evidence for current practice questioned
	Quality concern (efficiency, effectiveness, timeliness, equity, patient-centeredness)
	Safety or risk management concerns
	Unsatisfactory patient, staff, or organizational outcomes
	Variations in practice compared with external organizations
	Variations in practice within the setting
Knowledge-focused	New sources of evidence
	Changes in standards or guidelines
	New philosophies of care
	New information provided by organizational standards committees

Practice problems may be based on recurring or priority issues within an organization or the identification of practice that has questionable benefits. Clinical questions can help nurses understand differences in outcomes between two patient populations. For example, why do some patients in the intensive care unit (ICU) develop ventilator-associated pneumonia, whereas other ICU patients do not? There may be a difference in practice among nurses, nursing units, or peers outside of the organization. The potential for problems to generate practice questions is limitless. When the team invests time and effort to answer important EBP questions, potential benefits accrue to patients, healthcare teams, and organizations, such as:

- Increased visibility of healthcare team members' leadership and contributions
- New levels of support from clinicians and organizational leaders
- Tangible quality and safety benefits to patients and families
- Value-based organizational outcomes

Articulating a robust problem statement provides a comprehensive understanding of the population of interest (e.g., patients, families, staff, and their characteristics) and how they are affected (e.g., morbidity, mortality, satisfaction). Precise descriptions clarify the scope and magnitude of the problem related to the outcome of interest. Discussion of the problem enables the interprofessional team to reflect, gather information, observe current practice, listen to clinicians, visualize how the process can be different or improved, and probe the description—together fostering a shared understanding. Proceeding without a clear problem statement can result in:

- EBP questions that do not address the problem
- Searches that are too broad and lead the team to review more evidence than is needed to answer the question
- Missing evidence that is important to answer the question
- Team frustration with the effectiveness of the EBP process

Teams can use several strategies to help define problems. For example, phrasing the problem statement in terms of the knowledge gap rather than the solution or asking clarifying questions (e.g., where, why, when, how) allows the team to probe deeper into the nature or root cause of the problem. Table 4.3 provides specific strategies for defining the problem and provides an example of each one. Time spent defining the problem clearly and concisely will facilitate the construction of a good EBP question.

Table 4.3 Strategies for Defining the EBP Problem

Strategy	Examples	Rationale
Phrase the problem statement in terms of the knowledge gap, not the solution.	Instead of: Potential solution *Patients need a better pain management strategy for the immediate post-discharge period.* State: Knowledge gap *Staff lack knowledge of the best strategies to manage patient pain immediate post-discharge total knee replacement.*	Allows the team to see other, potentially more effective, solutions
State the problem rather than the symptoms of the problem.	Instead of: Symptom *Patients with total knee replacement were not satisfied after discharge.* State: Problem *40% of patients discharged post total knee replacement complain that they were not able to manage their pain.*	Allows the team to determine the true problem, and its size and scope, without being sidetracked by outward signs that a problem exists

continues

Table 4.3 Strategies for Defining the EBP Problem (cont.)

Strategy	Examples	Rationale
Describe in precise terms the perceived gap between what one sees and what one wants to see.	Gap: *Patient satisfaction with pain management post-discharge is 36%.* Aim: *Compare to a national benchmark of 85%.*	Allows the team to assess the current state and envision a future state in which broken components are fixed, risks are prevented, new evidence is accepted, and things that were missing elements are provided
Examine the problem critically, and make sure that the final statement defines the specific problem.	Instead of sticking with assumptions: Assumed problem *Are patients following the prescribed pain management regimen?* Identify a specific problem: *Do patients understand their pain management regimen?*	Gives the team time to gather information, observe, listen, and probe to ensure a true understanding of the problem
Ask clarifying questions.	Clarifying questions: *When are these patients experiencing pain? What are the precipitating factors? How often are they taking their pain medications?*	Helps the team get to the specific problem by using question words such as *when, what, how*
Refrain from blaming the problem on external forces or focusing attention on the wrong aspect of the problem.	Avoid attributing blame such as: *The patients are noncompliant with the prescribed pain-medication therapy. The nurses did not educate the patient properly about the importance of taking pain medications as prescribed.*	Keeps the team focused on processes and systems as the team moves to define the EBP question

State the problem differently.	Restating problem Revise from this: *40% of patients discharged post total knee replacement complained that they were not able to manage their pain.* To this: *40% of patients with post total knee replacement reported low patient satisfaction scores related to pain management after discharge.*	Helps gain clarity by using different verbs
Challenge assumptions.	Is the team's assumption correct? *The patient fills the pain medication prescription and is taking pain medication in the way that it was prescribed.*	Helps the team avoid conjecture and question everyday processes and practices that are taken for granted
Expand and contract the problem.	Expanded problem: *Is dissatisfaction with post-discharge pain management part of general dissatisfaction with the hospital stay as a whole?* Contracted problem: *Are there multiple reasons for dissatisfaction with post-discharge pain management, such as the inability to pay for pain medications or fear of becoming dependent on pain medications?*	Helps the team understand whether the problem is part of a larger problem or is made up of many smaller problems
Assume multiple solutions.	Single solution *What **is** the best practice for managing post-discharge pain in patients following total knee replacement?* Versus: Multiple solutions *What **are** the best practices for managing post-discharge pain in patients following total knee replacement?*	Helps the team identify more than one possible solution to determine the best fit for the population of interest

Developing and Refining the EBP Question

Having agreed on the nature and scope of the practice problem, the EBP team develops an answerable question that addresses a clinical, administrative, or knowledge problem. See Question Development Tool (Appendix B).

Choosing a Background or Foreground Question

There are two types of EBP questions: background and foreground (Sackett et al., 1996, 2000).

A *background question* is a best practice question that is broad and produces a wide range of evidence for review. EBP teams use background questions to identify and understand what is known when the team has little knowledge, experience, or expertise in the area of interest. For example, to better understand pain management for people with a history of substance abuse, a background question is: *What are the best interventions to manage pain for adult patients with a history of substance abuse enrolled in outpatient rehabilitation?* This question would produce an array of evidence, for example, pharmacology, alternative therapies, behavioral contracting, or biases in prescribing and administering pain medication. Evidence identified for background questions often provides a large number of results with diverse populations, settings, and interventions.

Foreground questions yield specific knowledge that informs decisions or actions and generally are used to compare two or more specific interventions. In some instances, the information gained from background questions informs the foreground questions. The following is an example of a foreground question: *Is behavioral contracting or mutual goal setting more effective in improving the chronic pain experience for adult patients enrolled in outpatient rehabilitation with a history of substance abuse?* Foreground questions produce a refined, limited body of evidence specific to the EBP question. In this example, the nature of pain is specified (chronic), and a comparison intervention is identified (mutual goal setting versus behavioral contracting).

One important point is when an EBP team is asking a background question, the evidence review can become complex. As a result, it may help organize the EBP project to break down the components of the problem into an appropriate number of background or foreground questions. To do this, the team could create questions that relate to each of the components identified during the initial evidence review. For example, to design a nursing preceptor program in a large health system, the EBP team posed this background question: *What are the best practices to train hospital-based nursing preceptors?* This question yielded a large amount of evidence that appeared to fall into three distinct categories: initial training, competencies, and ongoing support. From this evidence review, the team developed three more targeted and manageable background questions:

- What are the best practices to develop hospital-based nursing preceptors?
- What are the best practices to provide ongoing support to hospital-based preceptors?
- What are the essential competencies for hospital-based nursing preceptors?

> Teams with little experience with a topic or condition will have more background questions, whereas teams with more experience with the condition will generally have more foreground questions. Often, EBP teams will benefit from a thorough understanding of an issue's background before diving into the more specific foreground issues. As their understanding and experience with the topic or issue expand, they move into more focused foreground questions.

Writing an Answerable EBP Question

The thoughtful development of a well-structured EBP question is vital because the question drives the strategies used to search for evidence. Making the EBP question as specific as possible helps to identify and narrow search terms, which, in turn, reduces time spent searching for relevant evidence and increases the likelihood of finding it. Creating a specific question focuses the EBP project and provides a sensitive evidence review that accurately addresses the problem and question. It is also useful for defining the target population, such as age, gender, ethnicity, diagnosis, and procedure.

In 1995, Richardson and colleagues published a now widely used format for constructing an answerable EBP question referred to as PICO—patient, population or problem, intervention, comparison, and outcome. The PICO format is broadly accepted as the standard for defining clinical questions for evidence-based practice by framing the problem clearly and facilitating evidence retrieval by identifying key search terms (McKenzie et al., 2019).

*P*atient, Population, or Problem

Describe the patient, population, or problem succinctly. Include the type of patient or population and the setting. Consider attributes such as age, gender, symptoms, and diagnosis (patient's problem).

*I*ntervention

The intervention can be a treatment; a clinical, educational, or administrative intervention; a structure or process (see Table 4.4); strategies for education or learning; or assessment approaches.

*C*omparison With Other Intervention(s)

Background questions do not include a comparison. Foreground questions include comparison(s) of one intervention to another. The comparison group may be an intervention identified in the literature or a current practice.

*O*utcomes

This component requires that the team select measures that indicate the level of success in achieving the desired change, improvement, or outcome(s). Measures can be structure, process, or outcomes. For example, an EBP team may be concerned with decreasing patient falls in the medical-surgical unit. The team may employ a structural measure of examining the number of available patient safety observers on the unit. A process measure might investigate nurses' compliance with routine fall risk assessments. Finally, an outcome measure may look at the frequency of falls on the unit.

Once the team selects what they will measure, the next step is to define how they will quantify it. For example, if the measure of interest is the outcome of patient falls, the team determines the procedure for quantifying falls by determining a *metric*. A *metric* is the degree to which a particular subject possesses the quality of interest. Typically, it is calculated as a rate or proportion using a numerator and denominator. For the outcome measure of patient falls, the metric would be the total number of falls (numerator) per 1,000 patient days (denominator).

Table 4.4   Definitions and Examples of Structure, Process, and Outcome Measures of Care

Concept	Definition	Examples
Structure	Attributes of the setting	Adequacy of facility, equipment, and staff Qualifications of staff Availability of resources Policies
Process	Any patient care activity or intervention	Hand washing, aseptic technique Triage algorithms in the emergency department Medication administration
Outcome	Effects of care on health status and populations	Quality of life Patient satisfaction Surgical site infection

Source: Donabedian, 1988

Table 4.5 provides an example using PICO to create a foreground question. The question is: For adult surgical inpatients between the ages of 20 and 50 with a peripheral intravenous catheter, does the use of saline to flush the peripheral IV maintain IV patency and decrease phlebitis over 48 hours when compared to heparin flushes?

Table 4.5   PICO Example of a Foreground Question

P—Patient, population, or problem	Adult surgical inpatients (patients), between the ages of 20 and 50 years old with a peripheral intravenous catheter (population)
I—Intervention	Use of saline flushes
C—Comparison	Use of heparin flushes for peripheral IV maintenance
O—Outcomes	Improvements in IV patency over 48 hours (process) and a decrease in the incidence of phlebitis by 10% (outcome)

Determining the Need for an EBP Project

Changing practice requires an investment of time and resources. EBP teams need to carefully consider the projects they choose to pursue. Ideally, teams select problems of importance to the organization, department, or unit. Problems that merit further investigation can be related to the potential for harm, reflect unsatisfactory system or process performance or patient/staff experience, deviate from established standards of care, or be associated with high resource use (e.g., staffing or costs). With the advent of value-based purchasing, healthcare teams and organizations are financially rewarded or penalized for performance on quality and safety outcomes, preventable adverse conditions, and costs. It is important to remember that not all EBP improvements create cost savings. However, projects may achieve an equally valuable outcome (e.g., decreased infection rates) that addresses the organizational mission (Cullen & Hanrahan, 2018). Thus, it is crucial that before beginning the EBP project, EBP teams consider and select problems that align with identified priorities within their practice area. Before embarking on an EBP project and committing the necessary time and resources, consider the following questions:

- Would the practice changes resulting from this project improve clinical or staff outcomes, unit structures or processes, or patient or staff satisfaction or engagement?
- Would they reduce the cost of care?

- Can potential practice changes be implemented given the current culture, practices, and organizational structure within the particular practice setting?

In addition to considering whether the problem and EBP question match organizational priorities, EBP teams should conduct a preliminary search for evidence. This search should include both internal and external resources. First, teams should do an inventory of projects undertaken in their organization. Perhaps others have addressed similar problems. Teams can save valuable time by exploring and learning from previous work. Next, teams conduct an external search for evidence that accomplishes two goals: 1) identify whether sufficient research evidence exists to move forward with the project and 2) determine whether a high-quality evidence synthesis currently exists that addresses the problem. Figure 4.2 outlines this process.

A quick search of the literature, including major databases, allows teams to determine the presence or absence of research evidence related to the identified problem. If the preliminary scan reveals a lack of research or other forms of evidence related to the problem, teams should consider whether a quality improvement or research study would be more appropriate to address the problem. Other options include maintaining the current organizational practice or investigating/confirming the community standard. Only when the initial search of the literature indicates that sufficient evidence is available should the team proceed with the EBP project.

In addition to the availability of sufficient research evidence, EBP teams should look specifically for a high-quality, current (within five years), and applicable systematic review, such as a Cochrane Review that addresses the problem. Systematic reviews aim to identify, evaluate, and summarize the findings of relevant research studies on a healthcare topic, making the evidence easily accessible to decision-makers. If a high-quality review exists, the EBP team determines whether it is sufficient to address the EBP problem. Keep in mind, findings in one population or setting may not be transferable to another, and the EBP team should assess the fit to their specific setting. If appropriate, the team does not need to conduct a full EBP project and could proceed to the translation phase of the PET process. If a systematic review or evidence synthesis does not exist or is not of high quality, the EBP team proceeds to the remaining steps of the EBP process.

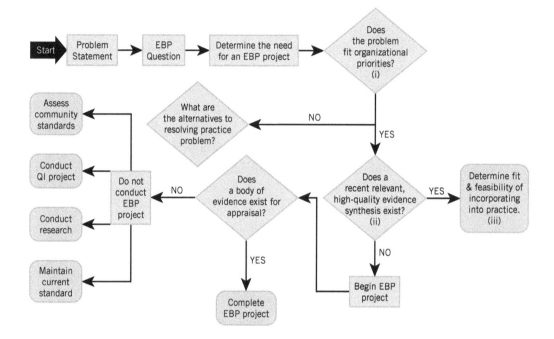

Key to the EBP Project Decision Tree:
i. Organizational priorities include unit, department, hospital, and programmatic.
ii. Team critically evaluates an existing evidence synthesis to ensure not only quality, but also that the findings are applicable to their setting and population and have been completed recently enough to represent the current environment. Make practice changes based only on high to moderate strength of syntheses of evidence, rather than on a single, low-quality evidence synthesis.
iii. Refer to the JHEBP Model and Guidelines for Nursing and Healthcare or the online EBP modules for assistance in determining fit, feasibility, and appropriateness.

Figure 4.2 Decision tree to determine the need for an EBP project.

Differentiating Between Quality Improvement, Research, and EBP

Before the discussion of EBP continues, it is important to consider EBP in the context of the three forms of inquiry. Differentiating between research, quality improvement (QI), and EBP can be challenging. Although QI, research, and EBP use distinctly different processes, commonalities among these three concepts include teamwork, critical thinking, and a commitment to improving care. The methods used and outcomes sought are different for each type of inquiry (see Table 4.6).

Table 4.6   Differentiating Between the Three Forms of Nursing Inquiry

	Quality Improvement	Research	Evidence-Based Practice
Starting point	A gap in performance of practice, process, or system	A gap in knowledge evidence	A gap in knowledge of best available evidence
Method	Plan-Do-Study-Act (PDSA), Six Sigma, Lean Principles	Scientific process	Practice Question, Evidence, Translation (PET) process
Outcome	Produces evidence for application at the local level (unit, department, organization)	Generates new knowledge for broad application	Synthesizes the best evidence for adoption in practice

Quality improvement is a process to improve healthcare services, systems, and processes at the local level (e.g., unit, department, organization) to improve outcomes (Jones, 2019). QI generally includes a method of measuring a particular outcome, making changes to improve practice and monitoring performance on an ongoing basis. QI may uncover a practice problem that initiates an EBP project. Some examples of QI initiatives are decreasing catheter-associated urinary tract infections, decreasing wait times in the emergency department, decreasing falls among patients, decreasing surgical site infections, improving patient satisfaction, improving pneumococcal and influenza immunization rates, and decreasing restraint use.

Research is a systematic investigation designed to develop, uncover, create, or contribute to new knowledge that can be generalized for broader application (US DHHS, 2018). It is often undertaken when no evidence or weak, conflicting, or incomplete evidence is returned during the search phase of an EBP project.

Research requires approval by an institutional review board (IRB) because the intent is to generalize knowledge beyond the usual care of the patient or setting. Research can impose additional risks or burdens not experienced in usual care, and the "subject" has the ethical right to decide whether they want to participate. Some examples of research are to create new evidence to compare pain management protocols on the experience of pain for ventilated patients; or evaluate two methods of communication (daily rounds conducted with clinicians only versus huddles incorporating patients and families) to compare satisfaction with patient engagement in decision-making for end-of-life care.

Evidence-based practice projects are undertaken when clinicians raise a concern or question important to practice that existing literature addresses. The EBP process starts with identifying a practice problem and reviewing the data or experience related to the problem; creating a specific question based on the identified problem; searching, retrieving, and reviewing the best available evidence; appraising the strength and quality of the retrieved evidence; synthesizing the quality, quality and consistency of the results; creating and implementing a translation to practice plan; and evaluating results and lessons learned. One example is exploring the literature to determine whether the use of plain disposable bathing wipes or traditional basin bathing represents the best practice to decrease the incidence of catheter-associated urinary tract infections (CAUTIs) because the evidence shows that wipes help. A second example is identifying best practices for improving patient safety and satisfaction on an inpatient oncology unit.

While these three forms of inquiry are distinct, they are linked when determining a course of action based on the nature of the question or problem raised by healthcare providers. As depicted in Figure 4.3, an interdisciplinary team raised the issue of increased infection rates in orthopedic patients with traction pins. Initially, efforts to decrease rates began as a QI project. On examining the current practice using the PDSA method, the team discovered that there was variation in pin care among the nurses. The team then undertook an EBP project to find the best available evidence on pin care. Finding no evidence in their search, they initiated a research study to generate new knowledge on the most effective pin care cleaning protocol for minimizing infection.

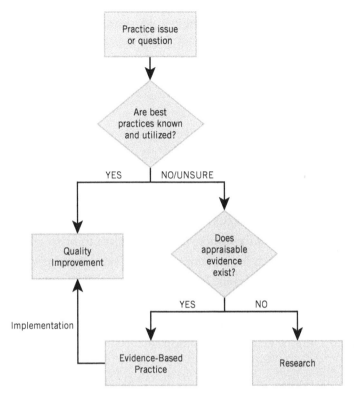

Figure 4.3 Choosing a form of inquiry for practice problems.

Identifying Stakeholders

After the team clarifies the problem and creates the EBP question, they reassess the need for stakeholders. A *stakeholder* is an individual or group who has an interest or "stake" in an activity or its evaluation (American Society for Quality, 2020). Team members may also fill the role of stakeholders. However, not all stakeholders are members of the EBP team. The EBP team needs to constantly assess the need for additional stakeholders. Stakeholders can affect the EBP project's outcome by supporting or limiting the translation of the project recommendations. The selection of appropriate stakeholders is based on who is affected by the problem or concern, where is it experienced, and when it occurs. Answering these questions influences who needs to be added to the team, informed, or involved. The project team should consider completing a stakeholder analysis matrix to ensure that all possible stakeholders are identified and ensure that appropriately identified communication strategies can be initiated with each one. *Note*: Consider involving a patient as a stakeholder or team member for patient-centered problems. Appendix C provides a stakeholder analysis matrix.

Summary

This chapter introduces the multiple sources of practice problems appropriate for an EBP approach. It is essential to begin this first stage of the EBP project systematically with an interprofessional team to define the problem and to generate an EBP question using the PICO format. EBP teams invest time to determine the need for an EBP project by comparing the problem to organizational priorities and conducting a search for existing evidence. Team members identify relevant stakeholders and their roles in the project. It is crucial to involve stakeholders early in the process to avoid delays and ensure success. The ultimate goal of the *P* phase in the PET process is a well-framed question to guide the next phase of the EBP process, the *E* (evidence) phase, successfully and efficiently.

References

American Society for Quality. (2020). *What are stakeholders?* https://asq.org/quality-resources/stakeholders

Cullen, L., & Hanrahan, K. (2018). *Evidence-based practice and the bottom line: An issue of cost.* Retrieved from https://www.hfma.org/topics/article/58754.html

Donabedian, A. (1988). The quality of care: How can it be assessed? *JAMA, 260,* 1743–1748. https://doi.org/10.1001/jama.260.12.1743

Institute of Medicine. (2003). *Health professions education: A bridge to quality.* The National Academies Press. https://doi.org/10.17226/10681

Institute of Medicine. (2013). *Interprofessional education for collaboration: Learning how to improve health from interprofessional models across the continuum of education to practice: Workshop summary.* The National Academies Press. https://doi.org/10.17226/13486

Jones, B., Vaux, E., & Olsson-Brown, A. How to get started in quality improvement. *BMJ* 2019; 364 :k5408 doi:10.1136/bmj.k5437

McKenzie, J. E., Brennan, S. E., Ryan, R. E., Thomson, H. J., Johnston, R. V., & Thomas J. (2019). Defining the criteria for including studies and how they will be grouped for the synthesis. In J. P. T. Higgins, J. Thomas, J. Chandler, M. Cumpston, T. Li, M. J. Page, & V. A. Welch (Eds.), *Cochrane handbook for systematic reviews of interventions,* version 6.0 (chapter 3). Cochrane. Available from https://training.cochrane.org/handbook/archive/v6/chapter-03

re:Work. (2020). *Guide: Understand team effectiveness.* https://rework.withgoogle.com/print/guides/5721312655835136/

Richardson, W. S., Wilson, M. C., Nishikawa, J., & Hayward, R. S. (1995). The well-built clinical question: A key to evidence-based decisions. *American College of Physicians, 123*(3), A12–A13.

Robert Wood Johnson Foundation. (2015). *Lessons from the field: Promising interprofessional collaboration practice.* https://www.michigan.gov/documents/mdch/Lessons_from_the_Field-Promising_Interprofessional_Collaboration_Practices_486256_7.pdf

Rogers, E. M. (2003). *Diffusions of innovations* (5th ed.). Free Press.

Sackett, D. L., Rosenberg, W. M., Gray, J. A., Haynes, R. B., & Richardson, W. S. (1996). Evidence based medicine: What it is and what it isn't. *British Medical Journal, 312*(7023), 71–72. https://doi.org/10.1136.bmj.312.7023.71

Sackett, D. L., Straus, S. E., Richardson, W. S., Rosenberg, W., & Haynes, R. B. (2000). *Evidence-based medicine: How to practice and teach EBM.* Churchill.

Titler, M. G., Kleiber, C., Steelman, V., Goode, C., Rakel, B., Barry-Walker, J., Small, S., & Buckwalter, K. (1994). Infusing research into practice to promote quality care. *Nursing Research, 43*(5), 307–313.

Titler, M. G., Kleiber, C., Steelman, V. J., Rakel, B. A., Budreau, G., Everett, L. Q., Buckwalter, K. C., Tripp-Reimer, T., & Goode, C. J. (2001). The Iowa model of evidence-based practice to promote quality care. *Critical Care Nursing Clinics of North America, 13*(4), 497–509.

US Department of Health and Human Services. (2018). *Code of Federal Regulations, Title 45 Public Welfare, Part 46 Protection of Human Subjects.* https://www.hhs.gov/ohrp/regulations-and-policy/regulations/45-cfr-46/index.html

Searching for Evidence

Information literacy is a set of abilities requiring individuals to "recognize when information is needed and have the ability to locate, evaluate, and use effectively the needed information" (American Library Association, 1989, para. 3). Developing information literacy skills requires knowledge of the nursing literature and an aptitude for locating and retrieving it. "Given the consistent need for current information in health care, frequently updated databases that hold the latest studies reported in journals are the best choices for finding relevant evidence to answer compelling clinical questions" (Fineout-Overholt et al., 2019, p. 60). Studies have shown that positive changes in a nurse's information literacy skills and increased confidence in using those skills have a direct impact on appreciation and application of research, are vital for effective lifelong learning, and are a prerequisite to evidence-based practice (McCulley & Jones, 2014).

EBP teams can collect evidence from a variety of sources, including the web and proprietary databases. The information explosion has made it difficult for healthcare workers, researchers, educators, administrators, and policymakers to process all the relevant literature available to them every day. Evidence-based clinical resources, however, have made searching for medical information much easier and faster than in years past. This chapter:

- Describes key information formats
- Identifies steps to find evidence to answer EBP questions
- Suggests information and evidence resources
- Provides tips for search strategies
- Suggests methods for screening and evaluating search results

Key Information Formats

Nursing, and healthcare in general, is awash with research data and resources in support of evidence-based nursing, which itself is continually evolving (Johnson, 2015). Evidence-based literature comes from many sources, and healthcare professionals need to keep them all in mind. The literature search is a vital component of the EBP process. If practitioners search only a single resource, database, or journal, they will likely miss important evidence. Likewise, target searching for a specific intervention or outcome may exclude important alternative perspectives. Through a thorough and unbiased search, healthcare professionals expand their experience in locating evidence important to the care they deliver.

Primary evidence is data generally collected from direct patient or subject contact, including hospital data and clinical trials. This evidence exists in peer-reviewed research journals, conference reports, abstracts, and monographs, as well as summaries from data sets such as the Centers for Medicare & Medicaid Services (CMS) Minimum Data Set. Databases that include primary source evidence include PubMed, Cumulative Index to Nursing and Allied Health Literature (CINAHL), the Cochrane Library, library catalogs, other bibliographic literature databases, and institutional repositories. For hospital administrators, the Healthcare Cost and Utilization Project (HCUP) is a source for health statistics and information on hospital inpatient and emergency department use.

Evidence summaries include systematic reviews, integrative reviews, meta-analysis, meta-synthesis, and evidence syntheses. The literature summaries that identify, select, and critically appraise relevant research use specific analyses to summarize the results of the studies. Evidence-based summaries also reside in library catalogs, online book collections, and online resources such as PubMed, CINAHL, the Cochrane Library, and JBI (formerly known as the Joanna Briggs Institute). For hospital administrators and case managers, Health Business Full Text is a source for quality improvement and financial information.

Translation literature refers to evidence-based research findings that, after much investigation and analysis, professional organizations or multi-disciplinary panels of experts translate for use in the clinical practice settings. Translation literature formats include practice guidelines, protocols, standards, critical pathways, clinical innovations, and evidence-based care centers and are available through peer-reviewed journals and bibliographic databases. JBI, CINAHL, and PubMed also provide this type of literature using Best Practice information sheets.

The Answerable Question

After identifying a practice problem and converting it into an answerable EBP question, the search for evidence begins with the following steps:

1. Identify the searchable keywords contained in the EBP question and list them on the Question Development Tool (see Appendix B). Include also any synonyms or related terms, and determine preliminary article inclusion criteria.

2. Identify the types of information needed to best answer the question, and list the sources where such information can be found. What database(s) will provide the best information to answer the question?

3. Develop a search strategy.

4. Evaluate search results for relevance to the EBP question.

5. Revise the search strategy as needed.

6. Record the search strategy specifics (terms used, limits placed, years searched) on the Question Development Tool and save the results.

7. Screen results to systematically include or exclude relevant literature.

EBP Search Examples

The first step in finding evidence is selecting appropriate search terms from the answerable EBP question. It may be useful to have a sense of the inclusion and exclusion criteria, which will guide the study selection. The Question Development Tool (Appendix B) facilitates this process by directing the team to identify the practice problem and, using the PICO components, to develop a searchable question.

For example, consider the following background question: What are best practices to reduce the rates of medical device-related pressure injuries in hospitalized adult patients? Some search terms to use may be *hospital, pressure injuries,* and *devices.* Table 5.1 illustrates how to use each part of an answerable PICO question to create an overall search strategy. Because the question addresses best practices that affect the outcomes, outcome search terms are not included in the search to avoid bias.

Table 5.1   PICO Example: Best Practices to Prevent Medical-Device Related Pressure Injuries

PICO Elements	Initial Search Terms	Related Search Terms
P: Adult hospitalized patients	*Inpatient* OR hospital**	*Ward OR unit OR floor OR nurs**
I: Best practices to prevent medical device-related pressure injuries	*Pressure injur* OR HAPI OR pressure ulcer* OR decubitis OR bedsore OR Braden scale*	*device OR devices OR tube OR tubes OR tubing OR catheter OR catheters OR nasal cannula* OR restraint* OR tape*

C: n/a

O: Rates of medical device-related pressure injuries

Table 5.2 displays another PICO question with each element mapped to potential search terms to help answer the EBP foreground question: In patients with chest tubes, does petroleum impregnated gauze reduce catheter dwell times as compared to a dry gauze dressing? In this case, the searcher may want to consider brand or product names to include in the search terms.

Table 5.2 PICO Example: Chest Tube Dressing Comparison

PICO Elements	Initial Search Terms	Related Search Terms
P: Patients with chest tubes	*Chest tube* OR chest drain**	*Pleural catheter* OR pleura shunt* OR intercostal drain OR (vendor-specific catheter names)*
I: petroleum impregnated gauze	*Petroleum*	*(vendor-specific name gauze) OR occlusive gauze*
C: dry gauze dressing	*Gauze*	*dressing OR bandage**
O: catheter dwell times	*dwell*	*Time OR hour* OR day**

Teams need to consider the full context surrounding the problem when thinking of search terms. As an example, *intervention* is a term used frequently in nursing; it encompasses the full range of activities a nurse undertakes in the care of patients. Searching the literature for nursing interventions, however, is far too general and requires a focus on specific interventions. Additionally, directional terms related to outcomes may bias the search. For example, including the term "reduce" will exclude potentially valuable information that may show alternative findings for the intervention in question.

Selecting Information and Evidence Resources

After selecting search terms, EBP teams can identify quality databases containing information on the topic. This section briefly reviews some of the unique features of core EBP databases in nursing and medicine.

CINAHL

CINAHL covers nursing, biomedicine, alternative or complementary medicine, and 17 allied health disciplines. CINAHL indexes more than 5,400 journals, contains more than 6 million records dating back to 1976, and has complete coverage of English-language nursing journals and publications from the National League for Nursing and the American Nurses Association (ANA). In addition, CINAHL contains healthcare books, nursing dissertations, selected conference proceedings, standards of practice, and book chapters. Full-text material within CINAHL includes more than 70 journals in addition to legal cases, clinical innovations, critical paths, drug records, research instruments, and clinical trials.

CINAHL also contains a controlled vocabulary, *CINAHL Subject Headings*, which allows for more precise and accurate retrieval. Selected terms are searched using "MH" for Exact Subject Heading or "MM" for Exact Major Subject Heading. Additionally, CINAHL allows searching using detailed filters to narrow results by publication type, age, gender, and language. The example PICO on pressure injuries could be searched using the CINAHL Headings. It may look like this:

> *(MH "Pressure Ulcer") AND (MH "Hospitalization" OR MH "Inpatients")*

MEDLINE and PubMed

MEDLINE and PubMed are often used interchangeably; however, teams need to keep in mind that they are *not* the same. PubMed is a free platform available through the National Library of Medicine's interface that searches not only MEDLINE but also articles not yet indexed in MEDLINE and articles that are included in PubMed Central.

MEDLINE, a database that contains over 30 million references (as of May 2020), includes journal articles in the life sciences with a concentration on biomedical research. One of MEDLINE's most notable features is an extensive, controlled vocabulary: *Medical Subject Headings (MeSH)*. An indexer, who is a specialist in a biomedical field, reviews each record in MEDLINE. The indexer assigns 5–15 appropriate MeSH terms to every record, which allows for precise searching and discovery. MeSH terms can help the searcher account for ambiguity and variations in spelling and language. A common saying in the library world is: "Garbage in, garbage out." MeSH terms can eliminate "garbage," or irrelevant articles. Searchers should be aware that not every record in PubMed receives MeSH indexing, so searching best practice involves including both MeSH terms and additional keywords for optimal evidence discovery.

To search in MEDLINE through PubMed using the PICO example for medical device-caused pressure injuries in hospitalized patients, one would use the MeSH term for *"Pressure Ulcer" [MeSH]* as the basis for the first concept. For the second concept, the searcher could select the MeSH terms *"Hospitalization"[MeSH]* and *"Inpatients"[MeSH]* to describe the concept of hospitalized patients, or alternatively, the MeSH term for *"Equipment and Supplies"[MeSH]*. There is no MeSH term for medical device, but *"equipment and supplies"* should capture some of that literature. A PubMed search strategy utilizing MeSH terms would look like this:

> *("Pressure Ulcer"[MeSH]) AND ("Hospitalization"[MeSH] OR "Inpatients"[MeSH])*

PubMed also contains *Clinical Queries*, a feature that has prebuilt evidence-based filters. *Clinical Queries* uses these filters to find relevant information on topics relating to one of five clinical study categories: therapy, diagnosis, etiology, prognosis, and clinical prediction guides. *Clinical Queries* also includes a search filter for systematic reviews. This filter adds predetermined limits to narrow the results to systematic reviews. To use the *Clinical Queries* feature, access it through the PubMed homepage, and enter the search as normal. *Clinical Queries* are beneficial only if a search has already been built.

The Cochrane Library

The Cochrane Library is a collection of databases that includes the Cochrane Database of Systematic Reviews. Internationally recognized as the gold standard in evidence-based healthcare, Cochrane Reviews investigate the effects of interventions for prevention, treatment, and rehabilitation. Over 7,500 Cochrane Reviews are currently available. Published reviews include an abstract, plain language summary, summaries of findings, and a detailed account of the review process, analysis, and conclusions. Abstracts of reviews are available free of charge from the Cochrane website; full reviews require a subscription. A medical librarian can identify an organization's access to this resource.

JBI (formerly known as the Joanna Briggs Institute)

JBI is an international, not-for-profit, membership-based research and development organization. Part of the Faculty of Health Sciences at the University of Adelaide, South Australia, JBI collaborates internationally with over 70 entities. The Institute and its collaborating entities promote and support the synthesis, transfer, and utilization of evidence by identifying feasible, appropriate, meaningful, and effective practices to improve healthcare outcomes globally. JBI includes evidence summaries and *Best Practice information sheets* produced specially for health professionals using evidence reported in systematic reviews. JBI resources and tools are available only by subscription through Ovid, and a medical librarian can identify an organization's access to this resource.

Selecting Resources Outside of the Nursing Literature

At times, it may become necessary to expand searches beyond the core nursing literature. Databases of a more general and multidisciplinary nature are presented in this section.

PsycINFO

PsycINFO is a database supported by the American Psychological Association that focuses on research in psychology and the behavioral and social sciences. PsycINFO contains more than 4.8 million records, including journal articles, book chapters, book reviews, editorials, clinical case reports, empirical studies, and literature reviews. The controlled vocabulary for PsycINFO is available through the Thesaurus feature. Users can search Thesaurus terms as major headings and explore terms to search for terms that are related and more specific. Users can limit searches in PsycINFO by record type, methodology, language, and age to allow for a more targeted search.

Health and Psychosocial Instruments (HaPI)

The HaPI database contains over 200,000 records for scholarly journals, books, and technical reports. HaPI, produced by the Behavioral Measurement Database Services, provides behavioral measurement instruments for use in the nursing, public health, psychology, social work, communication, sociology, and organizational behavior fields.

Physiotherapy Evidence Database (PEDro)

PEDro is a free resource that contains over 45,000 citations for randomized trials, systematic reviews, and clinical practice guidelines for physiotherapy. The Center for Evidence-Based Physiotherapy at the George Institute for Global Health produces this database and attempts to provide links to full text, when possible, for each citation in the database.

Creating Search Strategies and Utilizing Free Resources

In the following section, we will cover the necessary components used to create a robust search strategy. Databases are unique, so the components to select when creating a search strategy will vary; not every search strategy will utilize every component. The end of this section includes a list of free, reliable resources with descriptions explaining the content available in each resource. Remember to check with a local medical library to see what additional resources may be available.

Key Components to Creating Search Strategies

After identifying appropriate resources to answer the question, the EBP team can begin to create a search strategy. Keep in mind that this strategy may need adjustment for each database. Begin by breaking the question into concepts, selecting keywords and phrases that describe the concepts, and identifying appropriate controlled vocabulary, if available. Use *Boolean operators* (*AND, OR,* and *NOT*) to combine or exclude concepts. Remember to include spelling variations and limits where necessary. Note the search strategy examples' search strategies for PubMed and CINAHL in the previous sections were created by combining the AND and OR Boolean operators.

Use OR to combine keywords and controlled vocabulary related to the same concept (example searches formatted for PubMed):

("Pressure Ulcer"[MeSH] OR "pressure ulcer*" OR "pressure injur*" OR "decubitis")

Use AND to combine two separate concepts:

("Pressure Ulcer"[MeSH] OR "pressure ulcer*" OR "pressure injur*" OR "decubitis")

AND

("Hospitalization"[MeSH] OR "Inpatients"[MeSH] OR "hospital*" OR "inpatient*")

Review the following steps to build a thorough search strategy:

1. Use a controlled vocabulary when possible.

    Controlled vocabularies are specific subject headings used to index concepts within a database. They are essential tools because they ensure consistency and reduce ambiguity where the same concept may have different names. Additionally, they often improve the accuracy of keyword searching by reducing irrelevant items in the retrieval list. Some well-known vocabularies are MeSH in MEDLINE (PubMed) and CINAHL Subject Headings in CINAHL.

2. Choose appropriate keywords for the search's concepts.

    Look at key articles to see how they use the terms that define the topics. Think of possible alternative spellings, acronyms, and synonyms. Remember that even within the English language, spelling variations in American and British literature exist. In British literature, *S*s often replace *Z*s, and *OU*s often replace *O*s. Two examples of this are *organisation* versus *organization* and *behaviour* versus *behavior*.

3. Use Boolean operators.

    Boolean operators are AND, OR, and NOT. Use OR to combine keywords and phrases with controlled vocabulary. Use AND to combine each of the concepts within the search. Use NOT to exclude keywords and phrases; use this operator with discretion to avoid excluding terms that are relevant to the topic. (See Table 5.3.)

4. Use filters where appropriate.

    Most databases have extensive filters. PubMed and CINAHL allow filtering by age, gender, species, date of publication, and language. The filter for publication types assists in selecting the highest levels of evidence: systematic reviews, meta-analyses, practice guidelines, randomized controlled trials, and controlled clinical trials. Apply filters carefully and with justification, because it is easy to exclude something important when too many filters are applied.

5. Revise the search.

    As the team moves through Steps 1–4, they are likely to find new terms, alternate spellings of keywords, and related concepts. Revise the search to incorporate these changes. The search is only complete when the team can answer the question. If given a previous search to update, the team may need to make revisions because terms may have changed over time, and new related areas of research may have developed.

Table 5.3 Using Boolean Operators

Boolean Operator	Venn Diagram	Explanation	Example
AND		Use AND to link ideas and concepts where you want to see both ideas or concepts in your search results. The area in gray on the diagram highlights the recall of the search when AND is used to combine words or concepts. As you can see, AND narrows the search.	*"pressure ulcer" AND "hospitalization"*
OR		Use OR between similar keywords, like synonyms, acronyms, and variations in spelling within the same idea or concept. The area in gray on the diagram highlights the recall of the search when OR is used to combine words or concepts. As you can see, OR broadens the search.	*"pressure ulcer" OR "pressure injury"*
NOT		NOT is used to exclude specific keywords from the search; however, you will want to use NOT with caution because you may end up missing something important. The area in gray on the diagram shows the search results that you will get when you combine two concepts using NOT. As you can see, NOT is used to make broad exclusions.	*"pressure injury" NOT "crush injury"*

Free Resources

Most databases require a paid subscription, but some are freely searchable online. Table 5.4 lists quality web resources available at no cost. Check the local medical or public library to see what is accessible. Many databases are available through multiple search platforms. For example, teams can search the MEDLINE database through PubMed, but it is also available through other vendors and their platforms, such as EBSCOhost, ProQuest, and Ovid. Medical librarians, knowledgeable about available resources and how to use their functions, can assist in the search for evidence and provide invaluable personalized instruction. Never be afraid to ask for help! The only foolish question is the one unasked.

Table 5.4 Free Online Resources

Resource	Focus	Website
PubMed	Biomedical Research	https://pubmed.ncbi.nlm.nih.gov
PubMed Central	Full-Text Biomedical Resources	https://www.ncbi.nlm.nih.gov/pmc
Sigma Repository	Research, Dissertations, and Conference Abstracts	https://www.sigmarepository.org
The Cochrane Collaboration	Systematic Reviews and Controlled Trials	https://www.cochranelibrary.com
TRIP Medical Database (Turning Research Into Practice)	Clinical Practice	https://www.tripdatabase.com
US Preventive Services Task Force (USPSTF)	Clinician and Consumer Information	http://www.uspreventiveservicestaskforce.org
ClinicalTrials.gov	Clinical Trials	https://clinicaltrials.gov

continues

Table 5.4 Free Online Resources (cont.)

Resource	Focus	Website
NIH RePORTER: Research Portfolio Online Reporting Tool	Federally Funded Research Projects	http://report.nih.gov
Google Scholar	Multidisciplinary Resources	http://scholar.google.com

The *Sigma Repository* (formerly the *Virginia Henderson Global Nursing e-Repository)* is a resource offered through the Honor Society of Nursing, Sigma Theta Tau International. It gives nurses online access to easily utilized and reliable information. Primary investigator contact information is also available for requests of full-text versions of studies. The Sigma Repository also provides a list of tools, instruments, and measurements useful to nurses.

The *TRIP Medical Database* is a clinical search engine designed to allow health professionals to rapidly identify the highest-quality evidence for clinical practice. It searches hundreds of evidence-based medicine and nursing websites that contain synopses, clinical answers, textbook information, clinical calculators, systematic reviews, and guidelines.

The *US Preventive Services Task Force (USPSTF),* created in 1984, is an independent, volunteer panel of national experts in prevention and evidence-based medicine. It works to improve health by making evidence-based recommendations on clinical preventive services such as screenings, counseling services, and preventive medications, drawing from preventive medicine and primary care including family medicine, pediatrics, behavioral health, obstetrics and gynecology, and nursing.

Clinical Trials.gov is a resource providing patients, healthcare professionals, researchers, and the public with access to publicly and privately supported clinical studies for a variety of health conditions and diseases. The National Library of

Medicine (NLM) and the National Institutes of Health (NIH) maintain this resource. The principal investigator (PI) of the clinical study updates and provides information on the studies included. Currently, ClinicalTrials.gov contains data from studies conducted in all 50 states and over 216 countries. Searchers can look for studies that are currently recruiting as well as completed clinical studies.

NIH *Research Portfolio Online Reporting Tool (RePORTER)* is a federal government database that lists biomedical research projects funded by the NIH as well as the Centers for Disease Control and Prevention (CDC), Agency for Healthcare Research and Quality (AHRQ), Health Resources and Services Administration (HRSA), Substance Abuse and Mental Health Services Administration (SAMHSA), and US Department of Veterans Affairs (VA). RePORTER allows extensive field searching, hit lists that can be sorted and downloaded in Microsoft Excel, NIH funding for each project (expenditures), and publications and patents that have acknowledged support from each project (results).

Google Scholar is not associated with a hospital or academic library. It is a search aggregator that returns open and subscription results, including grey literature, such as conference proceedings, white papers, unpublished trial data, government publications and reports, and dissertations and theses. Google Scholar allows a broad search across many disciplines, searching academic publishers, professional societies, online repositories, universities, and other websites for articles, theses, books, abstracts, and court opinions. Searches can include non-medical terms, and due to its multidisciplinary nature, content can be accessed related to non-nursing subject matter. Google Scholar ranks documents by weighting the full text, publisher, and author(s), as well as how recently and frequently they are cited in other scholarly literature.

Though Google Scholar can be simple to use because of its familiarity and the wide use of Google as a search engine, the EBP team must be cautious. Search algorithms change daily, but journals are not indexed, making it impossible to replicate a search. As with a database, the EBP team must realize that searching using only Google Scholar will result in insufficient evidence (Gusenbauer &

Haddaway, 2020). With these caveats in mind, the EBP team can reap some additional benefits when using Google Scholar:

- A helpful feature is the user's ability to set up a Google Scholar profile, from which routine alerts for relevant search terms can be set up and sent via email notification. For example, if the EBP team is searching the literature using search terms *fall risk* and *acute care*, a recommendation rule can be set up so that any time Google adds a new document, an email can be sent directly to the EBP team, alerting them to this information.

- Google Scholar has the ability to both generate citations as well as export citations to citation managers to help keep track of references. By clicking on the closed quotation icon (") under a citation record, a pop-up will appear with a citation for the relevant document in a variety of output styles. Teams can directly copy or export these citations into a citation manager.

- Another benefit in Google Scholar is the "cited by" feature. By clicking on this option, Google Scholar will display publications that have cited the selected piece of literature. This can be helpful when trying to identify recent literature or other articles that may have used similar methods.

Additional Search Techniques

It is important to note that not all literature is found through database searching, either due to indexing or because the results were presented as a conference paper or poster and therefore not found in most databases. Because of this, the team can gain valuable information by:

- Hand searching the table of contents of subject-related, peer-reviewed journals, and conference proceedings
- Evaluating the reference list of books and articles cited in the eligible articles
- Searching for references citing relevant articles and evaluating the reference lists

Screening, Evaluating, Revising, and Storing Search Results

Whether EBP team members conduct a search independently or with the help of a medical librarian, it is the searchers' responsibility to evaluate the results for relevance based on the practice question as well as inclusion and exclusion criteria. Keep in mind that to answer the question thoroughly, a team's search strategies may need several revisions, and they should allow adequate time for these alterations.

When revising a search, consider these questions:

- *When was the last search conducted?* If the search is several years old, you need to consider changes that may have happened in the field that were missed by the previous search.
- *Have new terms been developed related to your search question?* Terms often change. Even controlled vocabulary such as MeSH is updated annually. Make sure to search for new controlled vocabulary and new keywords.
- *Did the search include databases beyond the nursing literature?* Are there databases outside of nursing that are relevant to your question? Does your question branch into psychology or physical therapy? Were those databases searched previously?
- *Are the limits used in the first search still appropriate?* If an age range limit was used in the last search, is it still relevant? Were there restrictions on publication type or methodology that are no longer useful?

After creating a successful search strategy, teams or individuals should keep a record of the work. Often individuals research the same topic throughout their career, so saving search strategies assists in updating work without duplication of effort. Most databases have a feature that allows saving a search within the database; however, it is always a good idea to keep multiple copies of searches. Microsoft Word documents or emails are a great way to keep a record of work.

PubMed is an example of a database that allows users to save multiple searches. *My NCBI*, a companion piece to PubMed, permits users to create an account, save searches, set alerts, and customize preferences. Users can save search results by exporting them into a citation management software program such as EndNote, RefWorks, Zotero, Mendeley, or Papers. Though some citation management programs are free, others need to be purchased; some may be provided at no cost by an organization. The function and capabilities of the various programs are similar.

Once the team downloads and stores search results, the next step is screening those results. Systematically and rigorously screening literature search results lends credence to the eventual recommendations from the project by ensuring a comprehensive and unbiased picture of the state of the evidence on a given topic, as well as saving time and effort among team members (Lefebvre et al., 2019; Whittemore & Knafl, 2005).

In addition to the question of rigor, comprehensive literature reviews can be a large undertaking with hundreds, if not thousands, of results. Screening is a necessary step to narrow the results of a search to only the pertinent results. It is important to note that a very large number of articles may be a sign that the search strategy or the practice question needs to be revised. Employing a team-based literature screening protocol and tracking mechanism helps to establish clear documentation of the process and makes screening more efficient and reliable. Following a step-wise approach of reviewing titles and abstracts, then full-text reading, conservatively allows a team to screen 500–1,000 articles over an eight-hour period (Lefebvre et al., 2019). Quickly culling superfluous results helps the team to home in on information truly relevant to the identified problem. With many competing priorities, EBP teams should avoid spending time considering articles that do not answer the EBP question through thoughtful approaches to the process.

The following steps outline how teams can create a well-documented literature screening process. These steps have been adapted from the *Cochrane Handbook for Systematic Reviews of Interventions* and the Preferred Reporting Items for

Systematic Reviews and Meta-Analyses (PRISMA) guidelines, which were created to improve reporting of systematic reviews (Lefebvre et al., 2019; Moher et al., 2009). While systematic reviews and EBP integrative reviews are different, they share the common goal of synthesizing the best evidence and are subject to similar risks. The EBP team meets to:

1. Establish inclusion and exclusion criteria for the literature screening.

   Commonly used exclusion criteria include population, language, date, intervention, outcomes, or setting. The team engages in critical thinking as they evaluate each article's potential contribution to answering the EBP question.

2. Establish a system (or way) for the EBP team to track the process for literature screening.

   If the team plans to publish their results, they may consider using tools such as Microsoft Excel to format search results and to function as a shared document for coding inclusion/exclusion. Including information related to the inclusion/exclusion criteria, duplicates removed, number of articles excluded at each stage, and any additional investigations outside of the systematic database search (e.g., hand searching) can strengthen the reporting of an EBP project. For systematic literature reviews, tools such as Covidence, Rayyan, and Abstrackr are available.

3. Decide how to complete the screening process.

   The literature screening process can be divided among all members of the EBP team. Best practice is to have at least two people review and agree whether an article should be included or excluded (Lefebvre et al., 2019; Polanin et al., 2019).

4. Begin by screening only the title and abstracts produced from the search.

   Performing a title screening and then returning to the remaining articles for an abstract screening can save time and distraction (Mateen et al., 2013). A key to remember in this step is that the article is included until proven otherwise. Exclude only those articles that concretely meet one of the exclusion criteria or do not answer the EBP question.

5. While screening, take notes.

   As the team delves deeper into the literature, they will gain a greater understanding of the available knowledge on a topic and the relevant vocabulary related to the practice question. Communicate as needed with the team members to make further group decisions on what to include and exclude in the search. There is no right or wrong answer; it is important that all group members have a common understanding of the scope of the project and that any changes or updates are well documented (de Souza et al., 2010).

6. After identifying citations, obtain full text.

   If full text is not available, submit the citation information through an interlibrary loan request with a local library. Prices associated with interlibrary loan vary with each library and each request. Contact a librarian for pricing inquiries. Some sites, such as EndNote Click and Unpaywall, can provide free, legal access to full text.

7. Complete full-text screening for all articles that remain after screening the titles and abstracts.

   Assigned reviewers complete a full-text reading of the articles to continue to determine whether they answer the EBP question and meet all inclusion criteria. This is an objective assessment and does not take into account the quality of the evidence. It is normal to continue to exclude articles throughout this stage.

Summary

This chapter illustrates how to use the PICO framework as a guide for literature searches. An essential component of evidence-based practice, the literature search is important to any research-and-publication activity because it enables the team to acquire a better understanding of the topic and an awareness of relevant literature. Information specialists, such as medical librarians, can help with complex search strategies and information retrieval.

Ideally, an iterative search process is used and includes: examining literature databases, using appropriate search terms, studying the resulting articles, and, finally, refining the searches for optimal retrieval. The use of keywords, controlled vocabulary, Boolean operators, and filters plays an important role in finding the most relevant material for the practice problem. Database alerting services are effective in helping researchers keep up to date with a research topic. Exploring and selecting from the wide array of published information can be a time-consuming task, so plan carefully in order to carry out this work effectively.

References

American Library Association. (1989). *Presidential committee on information literacy: Final report*. http://www.ala.org/acrl/publications/whitepapers/presidential

de Souza, M. T., da Silva, M. D., & de Carvalho, R. (2010). Integrative review: What is it? How to do it? *Einstein (São Paulo)*, 8(1), 102–106. https://doi.org/10.1590/S1679-45082010RW1134

Fineout-Overholt, E., Berryman, D. R., Hofstetter, S., & Sollenberger, J. (2019). Finding relevant evidence to answer clinical questions. In B. Mazurek Melnyk, & E. Fineout-Overholt (Eds.), *Evidence-based practice in nursing & healthcare: A guide to best practice* (pp. 36–63). Wolters Kluwer Health.

Gusenbauer, M., & Haddaway, N. R. (2020). Which academic search systems are suitable for systematic reviews or meta-analyses? Evaluating retrieval qualities of google scholar, PubMed, and 26 other resources. *Research Synthesis Methods*, 11(2), 181–217. https://doi.org/10.1002/jrsm.1378

Johnson, J. H. (2015). Evidence-based practice. In M. J. Smith, R. Carpenter, & J. J. Fitzpatrick (Eds.), *Encyclopedia of nursing education* (1st ed.), (pp. 144–146). Springer Publishing Company, LLC.

Lefebvre, C., Glanville, J., Briscoe, S., Littlewood, A., Marshall, C., Metzendorf, M. I., Noel-Storr, A., Rader, T., Shokraneh, F., Thomas, J., & Wieland, L. S. (2019). Searching for and selecting studies. In *Cochrane handbook for systematic reviews of interventions* (pp. 67–107). https://training.cochrane.org/handbook/current/chapter-04#section-4-6-5

Mateen, F., Oh, J., Tergas, A., Bhayani, N., & Kamdar, B. (2013). Titles versus titles and abstracts for initial screening of articles for systematic reviews. *Clinical Epidemiology*, 5(1), 89–95. https://doi.org/10.2147/CLEP.S43118

McCulley, C., & Jones, M. (2014). Fostering RN-to-BSN students' confidence in searching online for scholarly information on evidence-based practice. *The Journal of Continuing Education in Nursing*, 45(1), 22–27. http://dx.doi.org/10.3928/00220124-20131223-01

Moher, D., Liberati, A., Tetzlaff, J., Altman, D. G., & the PRISMA Group. (2009). Preferred reporting items for systematic reviews and meta-analyses: The PRISMA statement. *PLOS Medicine*, *6*(7), e1000097. https://doi.org/10.1371/journal.pmed.1000097

Polanin, J. R., Pigott, T. D., Espelage, D. L., & Grotpeter, J. K. (2019). Best practice guidelines for abstract screening large-evidence systematic reviews and meta-analyses. *Research Synthesis Methods*, *10*(3), 330–342. https://doi.org/10.1002/jrsm.1354

Whittemore, R., & Knafl, K. (2005). The integrative review: Updated methodology. *Journal of Advanced Nursing*, *52*(5), 546–553. https://doi.org/10.1111/j.1365-2648.2005.03621.x

Evidence Section

Introduction

Evidence hierarchies, one element used to determine best evidence, have been a tool of evidence-based healthcare for over 40 years (Burns et al., 2011). International groups, such as the Cochrane Library, World Health Organization (WHO), JBI, and the Agency for Healthcare Research and Quality (AHRQ) develop and apply evidence hierarchies to generate evidence-based recommendations (AHRQ, 2020; Higgins & Green, 2011; Pearson, 2005; WHO, 2012). Although there are dozens of classification systems, the overall goal is the same—to provide guidance on identifying the best evidence to change or improve practice.

Finding and evaluating evidence, the cornerstone of evidence-based healthcare, is the second phase in the JHEBP PET process. Evidence hierarchies are a tool to rank evidence according to the rigor of the methods of the evidence under review. This system puts evidence into tiered levels and allows for a shared understanding of how to evaluate and compare each piece of literature. Once the team determines the level of evidence, they assess the quality of the evidence appropriate for the specific method used. While the type of evidence governs the *level*, *quality* speaks to the execution and reporting of the review. This combination of *level* and *quality* yields an overall determination of the *strength* of the evidence, which is essential to generate sound recommendations and eventual translation to practice. The Johns Hopkins Evidence-Based Practice Model and Guidelines use a five-level evidence hierarchy. This is unique in that it includes not only research evidence (Levels I, II, and III), but nonresearch evidence as well (Levels IV, V). Figure E.1 displays the JHEBP evidence hierarchy.

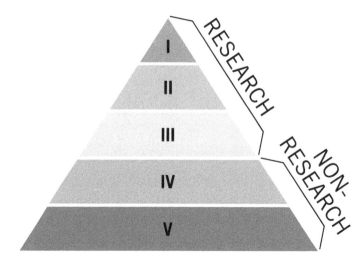

Figure E.1 Johns Hopkins Evidence-Based Practice evidence hierarchy.

Determining the level of evidence allows the team to complete the quality assessment using a corresponding quality scale. Rating scales assist in the critical appraisal of evidence by presenting a structured way to differentiate evidence of varying levels and quality. The Johns Hopkins model uses a three-point rating scale to give a grade of A ("high" quality), B ("good" quality), or C ("low" quality). Evidence with a rating of C is not included in the evidence summary and synthesis because the quality level is inadequate to generate reliable recommendations.

Within the JHEBP Model, determining the correct level of evidence is paramount, as it will direct you to the appropriate quality appraisal tool for Research Evidence (Appendix E) or Nonresearch Evidence (Appendix F). These lead the team through a series of "yes" or "no" questions to aid in critically evaluating an article. The Hierarchy of Evidence Guide (Appendix D) provides an overview of types of literature and specifies where they fall in the schema. Differentiating between types of evidence is a learned skill and improves with direct practice. EBP teams should use caution in taking evidence at face value because some terms are used interchangeably. This is especially true when differentiating research from quality improvement. See the "Differentiating Research from Quality Improvement" sidebar that follows. However, continue to evaluate whether elements such as approval, consent, and opting-in or -out were not included because the project is in fact quality improvement, rather than a poorly executed or reported on research study.

Differentiating Research (Levels I-III) from Quality Improvement (Level V) Evidence

- All research requires ethical approval. For research, the methods section of an article should speak to the ethical (also known as the Institutional Review Board; IRB) approval process. If there is no mention of ethical review, it is unlikely the evidence is research. If the report mentions ethical approval, read carefully to see what the review board determined as the project category. Some institutions also submit QI projects to the IRB, and the designation as QI should be noted.

- Research also requires consent (either implied or explicit). If there is no mention of obtaining consent, the project is unlikely to be research.

- Similar to consent, research also must give people the opportunity to opt in or opt out of participation. If a project describes a broad intervention (sometimes a process change or change to the standard of care) that affected all participants without the ability to decline, the project is more likely to be quality improvement. For example, if a unit has decided to use a new staffing model for ALL providers, this is more likely quality improvement, as staff do not have the opportunity to opt in or out of the new process.

Evidence Summary

As the members of the EBP team read each of the articles that answer the EBP question, they begin to collate that information in the Individual Evidence Summary Tool (Appendix G). In larger EBP projects, it is not feasible to have every team member read every article. It is preferable that teams assign two independent reviewers to complete the evidence appraisal to ensure accuracy. The individual evidence summary provides a centralized document the whole team can use to record and share the pertinent information for each of their assigned articles. Ideally, the reviewers provide sufficient information so that the other team members understand the key findings of the article without needing to go to the source material. The individual evidence summary table provides headers to guide the team through the data entry process. When possible, at least two reviewers should appraise each article and reach a consensus on both the level and the quality. In addition to having a group understanding of the type of information entered into the table, it may also be beneficial to discuss any additional elements the team would like to track and record these in the "notes" column. Once complete, the team sorts the articles by level and quality. Low-quality articles are not included in the subsequent steps of the EBP process.

Of note, EBP teams should be attentive to identify duplicate publications—that is, more than one publication that reports findings from the same research study, such as a primary research study that is then included in a subsequent literature review or an expert's opinion of an organization's position statement. This may result in a distortion of the available evidence due to an overrepresentation of data from one source. There is no standard protocol to address this type of duplicative information, and the team should discuss how to handle repetitions on a case-by-case basis.

Evidence Synthesis

After the team collates all of the "good" and "high" quality evidence in the Individual Evidence Summary Tool (Appendix G), the team uses this document to synthesize the findings at each level and generate best practice recommendations through critical thinking using the Synthesis and Recommendations Tool (Appendix H).

Synthesis is the process of combining two or more elements to create a new idea or understanding, with the whole being greater than the sum of its parts. This means the literature synthesis is not a repetition of the data points in the individual evidence summary but rather the creation of an overall picture of the body of the evidence. Synthesis generates new insights, perspectives, and understandings through group discussion and consensus building through each of the levels of evidence.

> **Summary vs. Synthesis: Clinical Example**
>
> Healthcare providers are well practiced at summarizing patient information and synthesizing that data to create an overall picture of the patient's condition. For example, a patient may have a fever, tachycardia, lethargy, hypotension, and pneumonia noted on their chest X-ray. This information provides individual data (individual evidence) about the patient, but the true takeaway (synthesis) is the patient has sepsis. Healthcare providers use clinical experience and critical thinking to move beyond listing data to create a greater understanding of the overall patient picture.

Just as determining a patient's diagnosis by synthesizing individual data points is an advanced skill for healthcare providers, so is interpreting individual evidence findings to determine how it contributes to answering the PICO question. Both require direct practice, experience, and critical thinking, and both benefit from mentorship. It can be beneficial to think about different aspects of the findings by sorting and assigning themes or labels. Additionally, comparing specific aspects of each article side by side may lend more significant insights (e.g., perhaps the intervention worked well with students, but not with post-licensure professionals; or audit and feedback improved performance with documentation, but not performing a skill).

Then the team uses the synthesis of each level of evidence to generate best evidence recommendations that take into account the 1) strength (level and quality) of evidence, 2) quantity of evidence, and 3) consistency of findings.

The strength and quantity of evidence is determined and recorded from the Individual Evidence Summary Tool (Appendix G). The consistency of findings requires an overall determination of the agreement of evidence findings within each level. Identifying points of consistency as well as inconsistency lends additional insights into the overall body of the evidence and how the evidence might contribute to best practice recommendations. In general, multiple high-quality studies of Level I and II evidence build confidence in recommendations. Teams do not make practice changes based on low-quality evidence or Level IV and V evidence alone. This step reflects the best overall evidence and does not yet take into account the practice setting of the EBP team. The Synthesis and Recommendations Tool (Appendix H) outlines the steps of this process and provides guidance on possible outcomes of an assessment of the evidence.

> **Clinical Example of Leveraging Data for Greater Understanding**
>
> A clinician has an inpatient's medication administration record and a vital sign documentation flowsheet. Putting this documentation side by side creates greater insights into both sets of data rather than if they were read alone. For example, a patient may exhibit hypoxia with improvement, followed by tachycardia. This information may cause concern if not layered with knowing that the patient received a breathing treatment with a side effect of elevated heart rate to resolve the low oxygen saturation. Examining and comparing specific data elements can be a powerful tool for a greater understanding of the larger picture.

Summary

The evidence portion of the EBP project is the crux of the EBP process. Without an in-depth understanding of best evidence related to the practice problem, organizational change can at best falter and at worst cause harm. Tools such as evidence hierarchies, appraisal tools, and collating tools create a common vocabulary and workflow among the EBP team to assess and report findings. Critical thinking and consensus building then transition repeated information into new meaning. A robust synthesis of best evidence recommendations with careful considerations and highly developed critical thinking can make a good

EBP project, a great EBP project. This builds a strong and reliable foundation for organizational translation, which builds on the process with the addition of clinical reasoning.

References

Agency for Healthcare Research and Quality. (2020). *EPC evidence-based reports*. https://www.ahrq.gov/research/findings/evidence-based-reports/index.html

Burns, P. B., Rohrich, R. J., & Chung, K. C. (2011). The levels of evidence and their role in evidence-based medicine. *Plastic and reconstructive surgery*, *128*(1), 305.

Higgins, J. P. T., & Green, S. (Eds.). (2011). *Cochrane handbook for systematic reviews of interventions* (5.1.0 ed.). http://handbook.cochrane.org

Pearson, A., Wiechula, R., Court, A., & Lockwood, C. (2005). The JBI model of evidence-based healthcare. *International Journal of Evidence-Based Healthcare*, *3*(8), 207–215.

World Health Organization. (2012). *WHO handbook for guideline development*. WHO Press.

Evidence Appraisal: Research

Evidence-rating schemes consider scientific evidence—also referred to as *research*—to be the strongest form of evidence. The underlying assumption is that recommendations from higher levels of high-quality evidence will be more likely to represent best practices. While comparatively stronger than nonresearch evidence, the strength of research (scientific) evidence can vary between studies depending upon the methods used and the quality of reporting by the researchers. The EBP team begins its evidence search in the hope of finding the highest level of scientific evidence available on the topic of interest.

This chapter provides:

- An overview of the various types of research approaches, designs, and methods
- Guidance on how to appraise the level and quality of research evidence to determine its overall strength
- Tips and tools for reading and evaluating research evidence

Types of Scientific Research

The goal of research is to produce new knowledge that can be generalized to a wider population by systematically following the scientific method. *Research approaches* are the general frameworks researchers use to structure a study and collect and analyze data (Polit & Beck, 2017). These fall in three broad categories: quantitative, qualitative, and mixed methods. Researchers use these approaches across the spectrum of research designs (e.g., experimental, quasi-experimental, descriptive), which primarily dictate the research methods used to gather, analyze, interpret, and validate data during the study. The chosen technique will depend on the research question as well as the investigators' background, worldviews (paradigms), and goals (Polit & Beck, 2017).

Quantitative Research

Most scientific disciplines predominantly use a quantitative research approach to examine relationships among variables. This approach aims to establish laws of behavior and phenomena that are generalizable across different settings and contexts. This research approach uses objective and precise collection such as observation, surveys, interviews, documents, audiovisuals, or polls to measure data quantity or amount. Through numerical comparisons and statistical inferences, data analysis allows researchers to describe, predict, test hypotheses, classify features, and construct models and figures to explain what they observe.

Qualitative Research

Qualitative research approaches, rooted in sociology and anthropology, seek to explore the meaning individuals, groups, and cultures attribute to a social or human problem (Creswell & Creswell, 2018). Thus, the researcher studies people and groups in their natural setting and obtains data from an informants' perspective. Using a systematic subjective approach to describe life experiences, qualitative researchers are the primary data collection instrument. By analyzing data, they attempt to make sense of or interpret phenomena in terms of the meanings people bring to them. In contrast to quantitative research, qualitative studies do not seek to provide representative data but rather information saturation.

Mixed-Methods Research

A mixed-methods research approach intentionally incorporates or "mixes" both quantitative and qualitative designs and data in a single study (Creswell & Creswell, 2018). Researchers use mixed methods to understand contradictions between quantitative and qualitative findings; assess complex interventions; address complex social issues; explore diverse perspectives; uncover relationships; and, in multidisciplinary research, focus on a substantive field, such as childhood depression.

Qualitative and quantitative research designs are complementary. However, while a quantitative study can include qualitative data, such as asking an open-ended question in a survey, it is not automatically considered to be mixed-methods because the design sought to address the research questions from a quantitative perspective (how many, how much, etc.). Likewise, a qualitative study may gather quantitative data, such as demographics, but only to provide further insights into the qualitative analysis. The research problem and question drive the decision to use a true mixed-methods approach and leverage the strengths of both quantitative and qualitative designs to provide a more in-depth understanding than either would if used independently. If using only quantitative or qualitative designs would provide sufficient data, then mixed methods are unnecessary.

Types of Research Designs

Research problems and questions guide the selection of a research approach (qualitative, quantitative, or mixed methods) and, within each approach, there are different types of inquiries, referred to as research designs (Creswell & Creswell, 2018). A research design provides specific direction for the methods used in the conduct of the actual study. Additionally, studies can take the form of single research studies to create new data (primary research), summarize and analyze existing data for an intervention or outcome of interest (secondary research), or represent summaries of multiple studies.

Single Research Studies

The evidence-based practice (EBP) team will typically review evidence from single research studies or primary research. Primary research comprises data collected to answer one or more research questions or hypotheses. Reviewers may also find secondary analyses that use data from primary studies to ask different questions. Single research studies fall into three broad categories: true experimental, quasi-experimental, and nonexperimental (observational).

Table 6.1 outlines the quantitative research design, aim, distinctive features, and types of study methods frequently used in social sciences.

Table 6.1 Research Design, Aim, Distinctive Features, and Types of Study Methods

Research Design	Aim	Features	Type of Study Methods
True Experimental	Establish existence of a cause and effect relationship between an intervention and an outcome	■ Manipulation of a variable in the form of an intervention ■ Control group ■ Random assignment to the intervention or control group	■ Randomized controlled trial ■ Posttest-only with randomization ■ Pre- and posttest with randomization ■ Solomon 4 group

Quasi-experimental	Estimate the causal relationship between an intervention and an outcome without randomization	■ An intervention
		■ Nonrandom assignment to an intervention group; may also lack a control group
			■ Nonequivalent groups: not randomized
			   ■ control (comparison) group posttest only
			   ■ pretest–posttest
			■ One group: not randomized
			   ■ posttest only
			   ■ pretest–posttest
			■ Interrupted time-series

Non-experimental	Measures one or more variables as they naturally occur without manipulation	▪ May or may not have an intervention ▪ No random assignment to a group ▪ No control group	▪ Descriptive ▪ Correlational ▪ Qualitative
Univariate	Answers a research question about one variable or describes one characteristic or attribute that varies from observation to observation	▪ No attempt to relate variables to each other ▪ Variables are observed as they naturally occur	▪ Exploratory ▪ Survey ▪ Interview

Source: Creswell & Creswell, 2018

True Experimental Designs (Level I Evidence)

True experimental studies use the traditional scientific method: independent and dependent variables, pretest and posttest, and experimental and control groups. One group (experimental) is exposed to an intervention; the other is not exposed to the intervention (the control group). This study design allows for the highest level of confidence in establishing causal relationships between two or more variables because the variables are observed under controlled conditions (Polit & Beck, 2017). True experiments are defined by the use of randomization. The most commonly recognized true experimental method is the randomized controlled trial, which aims to reduce certain sources of bias when testing the effectiveness of new treatments and drugs. However, other methods of true experimental designs that require randomization are listed in Table 6.1. The

Solomon 4 group is frequently used in psychology and sometimes used in social sciences and medicine. It is used specifically to assess whether taking a pretest influences scores on a posttest.

A true experimental study has three distinctive criteria: *randomization, manipulation*, and *control.*

Randomization occurs when the researcher assigns subjects to a control or experimental group arbitrarily, similar to the roll of dice. This process ensures that each potential subject who meets inclusion criteria has the same probability of selection for the experiment. The goal is that people in the experimental group and the control group generally will be similar, except for the experimental intervention or treatment. This is important because subjects who take part in an experiment serve as representatives of the population, and as little bias as possible should influence who does and does not receive the intervention.

Manipulation occurs when the researcher implements an intervention with at least some of the subjects. In experimental research, some subjects (the *experimental group*) receive an intervention and other subjects do not (the *control group*). The experimental intervention is the *independent variable,* or the action the researcher will take (e.g., applying low-level heat therapy) to try to change the *dependent variable* (e.g., the experience of low back pain).

Control usually refers to the introduction of a control or comparison group, such as a group of subjects to which the experimental intervention is *not* applied. The goal is to compare the effect of no intervention on the dependent variable in the control group against the experimental intervention's effect on the dependent variable in the experimental group. Control groups can be achieved through various approaches and include the use of placebos, varying doses of the intervention between groups, or providing alternative interventions (Polit & Beck, 2017).

> **Example: Experimental Randomized Controlled Trial**
>
> Rahmani et al. (2020) conducted a randomized control trial to investigate the impact of Johnson's Behavioral System Model in the health of heart failure patients. They randomized 150 people to a control group and an intervention group. The intervention group received care based on findings from a behavioral subsystem assessment tool, and the control group received care based on their worst subsystem scores over a two-week period. The researchers found that the intervention group showed significant improvement in six of the eight subsystems over the control group.

Quasi-Experimental Designs (Level II Evidence)

Quasi-experimental studies are similar to experimental studies in that they try to show that an intervention causes a particular outcome. Quasi-experimental studies always include manipulation of the independent variable (intervention). They differ from true experimental studies because it is not always possible to randomize subjects, and they may or may not have a control group. For example, an investigator can assign the intervention (manipulation) to one of two groups (e.g., two medical units); one unit volunteers to pilot a remote video fall reminder system (intervention group) and is compared to the other unit that continues delivering the standard of care (control group). Although the preexisting units were not randomly assigned, they can be used to study the effectiveness of the remote video reminder system.

In cases where a particular intervention is effective, withholding that intervention would be unethical. In the same vein, it may not be feasible to randomize patients or geographic location, or it would not be practical to perform a study that requires more human, financial, or material resources than are available.

Examples of types of important and frequently used quasi-experimental designs that an EBP team may see during the course of their search include nonequivalent control (comparison), one group posttest only, one group pretest–posttest, and interrupted time series design. The EBP team members should refer to a research text when they encounter any unfamiliar study designs.

> **Examples: Quasi-Experimental Studies**
>
> Awoke et al. (2019) conducted a quasi-experimental study to evaluate the impact of nurse-led heart failure patient education on knowledge, self-care behaviors, and all cause 30-day hospital readmission. The study used a pretest and posttest experimental design on a convenience sample in two cardiac units. An evidence-based education program was developed based on guidelines from the American Colleges of Cardiology and American Heart Association. Participants were invited to complete two validated scales assessing heart failure knowledge and self-care. The researchers found a statistically significant difference in knowledge and self-care behaviors. A significant improvement in 30-day readmission was not found.

Nonexperimental Designs (Level III Evidence)

When reviewing evidence related to healthcare questions, EBP teams will often find studies of naturally occurring phenomena (groups, treatments, and individuals), situations, or descriptions of the relationship between two or more variables. These studies are nonexperimental because there is no interference by the researcher. This means that there is no manipulation of the independent variable or random assignment of participants to a control or treatment group, or both. Additionally, the validity of measurements (e.g., physiologic values, survey tools), rather than the validity of effects (e.g., lung cancer is caused by smoking), is the focus of attention.

Nonexperimental studies fall into three broad categories—descriptive, correlational, and qualitative univariate (Polit & Beck, 2017)—and can simultaneously be characterized from a time perspective. In *retrospective* studies, the outcome of the study has already occurred (or has not occurred in the case of the controls) in each subject or group before they are asked to enroll in the study. The investigator then collects data either from charts and records or by obtaining recall information from the subjects or groups. In contrast, for *prospective* studies, the outcome has not occurred at the time the study begins, and the investigator follows up with subjects or groups over a specific period to determine the occurrence of outcomes. In *cross-sectional* studies, researchers collect data from many different individuals at a single point in time and observe the variables of interest without influencing them. *Longitudinal* studies look at changes in the same subjects over a long period.

Descriptive Studies

Descriptive studies accurately and systematically describe a population, situation, or phenomenon as it naturally occurs. It answers what, where, when, and how questions but does not answer questions about statistical relationships between variables. There is no manipulation of variables and no attempt to determine that a particular intervention or characteristic causes a specific occurrence to happen. Answers to descriptive research questions are objectively measured using statistics, and analysis is generally limited to measures of frequency (count, percent, ratios, proportions), central tendency (mean, median, mode), dispersion or variation (range, variance, standard deviation), and position (percentile rank, quartile rank). A descriptive research question primarily quantifies a single variable but can also cover multiple variables within a single question. Common types of descriptive designs include descriptive comparative, descriptive correlational, predictive correlational, and epidemiologic descriptive studies (prevalence and incidence). Table 6.2 outlines the purpose and uses of quantitative descriptive design study types.

Table 6.2 Descriptive Study Type, Purpose, and Use

Descriptive Study Type	Purpose	Use
Comparative	Determine similarities and difference or compare and contrast variables without manipulation.	Account for differences and similarities across cases; judge if a certain method, intervention, or approach is superior to another.
Descriptive correlational	Describe two variables and the relationship (strength and magnitude) that occurs naturally between them.	Find out if and how a change in one variable is related to a change in the other variable(s).
Incidence (epidemiologic descriptive)	Determine the occurrence of new cases of a specific disease or condition in a population over a specified period of time.	Understand the frequency of new cases for disease development.

continues

Table 6.2   Descriptive Study Type, Purpose, and Use (cont.)

Descriptive Study Type	Purpose	Use
Predictive correlational	Predict the variance of one or more variables based on the variance of another variable(s).	Examine the relationship between a predictor (independent variable) and an outcome/criterion variable.
Prevalence (epidemiologic descriptive)	Determine the proportion of a population that has a particular condition at a specific point in time.	Compare prevalence of disease in different populations; examine trends in disease severity over time.

Correlational Studies

Correlational studies measure a relationship between two variables without the researcher controlling either of them. These studies aim to find out whether there is:

- *Positive* correlation: One variable changes in the same direction as the other variable direction.
- *Negative* correlation: Variables change in opposite directions, one increases, and the other decreases.
- *Zero* correlation: There is no relationship between the variables.

Table 6.3 outlines common types of correlational studies, such as case-control, cohort, and natural experiments.

Table 6.3 Correlational Study Type, Purpose, and Use

Correlational Study Type	Purpose	Use
Case-control	Examine possible relationships between exposure and disease occurrence by comparing the frequency of exposure of the group with the outcome (cases) to a group without (controls). Can be either retrospective or prospective.	Identifies factors that may contribute to a medical condition. Often used when the outcome is rare.
Cohort	Examine whether the risk of disease was different between exposed and nonexposed patients. Can be either retrospective or prospective.	Investigates the causes of disease to establish links between risk factors and health outcomes.
Natural experiments	Study a naturally occurring situation and its effect on groups with different levels of exposure to a supposed causal factor.	Beneficial when there has been a clearly defined exposure involving a well-defined group and the absence of exposure in a similar group.

Univariate Studies

Univariate studies, also referred to as single-variable research, use exploratory or survey methods and aim to describe the frequency of a behavior or an occurrence. Univariate descriptive studies summarize or describe one variable, rather than examine a relationship between the variables (Polit & Beck, 2017). Exploratory and survey designs are common in nursing and healthcare. When little knowledge about the phenomenon of interest exists, these designs offer the greatest degree of flexibility. Though new information is learned, the direction of the exploration may change. With exploratory designs, the investigator does not know enough about a phenomenon to identify variables of interest completely. Researchers observe variables as they happen; there is no researcher control. When investigators know enough about a particular phenomenon and can identify specific variables of interest, a descriptive survey design more fully describes the phenomenon. Questionnaire (survey) or interview techniques assess the variables of interest.

Qualitative Research Designs

Qualitative research designs seek to discover the whys and hows of a phenomenon of interest in a written format as opposed to numerical. Types of qualitative studies (sometimes referred to as traditions) include ethnography, grounded theory, phenomenology, narrative inquiry, case study, and basic qualitative descriptive. With the exception of basic qualitative descriptive, each study type adheres to a specific method for collecting and analyzing data; each methodology is based upon the researcher's worldview that consists of beliefs that guide decisions or behaviors. Table 6.4 details qualitative study types.

Table 6.4 Qualitative Study Type, Purpose, Uses

Type	Purpose	Use
Ethnography	Study of people in their own environment to understand cultural rules	Gain insights into how people interact with things in their natural environment.
Grounded theory	Examine the basic social and psychological problems/concerns that characterize real-world phenomena	Used where very little is known about the topic to generate data to develop an explanation of why a course of action evolved the way it did.
Phenomenology	Explore experience as people live it rather than as they conceptualize it	Understand the lived experience of a person and its meaning.
Narrative inquiry	Reveal the meanings of individuals' experiences combined with the researcher's perspective in a collaborative and narrative chronology	Understand the way people create meaning in their lives.

Case study	Describe the characteristics of a specific subject (such as a person, group, event, or organization) to gather detailed data to identify the characteristics of a narrowly defined subject	Gain concrete, contextual, in-depth knowledge about an unusual or interesting case that challenges assumptions, adds complexity, or reveals something new about a specific real-world subject.
Basic qualitative (also referred to as *generic* or *interpretive descriptive*)	Create knowledge through subjective analysis of participants in a naturalistic setting by incorporating the strengths of different qualitative designs without adhering to the philosophical assumptions inherent in those designs	Problem or phenomenon of interest is unsuitable for, or cannot be adapted to, the traditional qualitative designs.

Systematic Reviews: Summaries of Multiple Research Studies

Summaries of multiple research studies are one type of evidence synthesis that generates an exhaustive summary of current evidence relevant to a research question. Often referred to as *systematic reviews*, they use explicit methods to search the scientific evidence, summarize critically appraised and relevant primary research, and extract and analyze data from the studies that are included in the review. To minimize bias, a group of experts, rather than individuals, applies these standardized methods to the review process. A key requirement of systematic reviews is the transparency of methods to ensure that rationale, assumptions, and processes are open to scrutiny and can be replicated or updated. A *systematic review* does not create new knowledge; rather, it provides a concise and relatively unbiased synthesis of the research evidence for a topic of interest (Aromataris & Munn, 2020).

There are at least 14 types of systematic review study designs (Aromataris & Munn, 2020) with specific critical appraisal checklists by specific study design type (Grant & Booth, 2009). Healthcare summaries of multiple studies most often use meta-analyses with quantitative data and meta-syntheses with qualitative data.

> **Systematic Reviews Versus Narrative Reviews**
>
> Systematic reviews differ from traditional narrative literature reviews. Narrative reviews often contain references to research studies but do not critically appraise, evaluate, and summarize the relative merits of the included studies. True systematic reviews address both the strengths and the limitations of each study included in the review. Readers should not differentiate between a systematic review and a narrative literature review based solely on the article's title. At times, the title will state that the article presents a literature review when it is in fact a systematic review or state that the article is a systematic review when it is a literature review. EBP teams generally consider themselves lucky when they uncover well-executed systematic reviews that include summative research techniques that apply to the practice question of interest.

Systematic Review With Meta-Analysis

Meta-analyses are systematic reviews of quantitative research studies that statically combine the results of multiple studies that have a common intervention (independent variables) and outcomes (dependent variables) to create new summary statistics. Meta-analysis offers the advantage of objectivity because the study reviewers' decisions are explicit and integrate data from all included studies. By combining results across several smaller studies, the researcher can increase the power, or the probability of detecting a true relationship between the intervention and the outcomes of the intervention (Polit & Beck, 2017).

For each of the primary studies, the researcher develops a common metric called effect size (ES), a measure of the strength of the relationship between two variables. This summary statistic combines and averages effect sizes across the included studies. Cohen's (1988) methodology for determining effect sizes defines the strength of correlation ratings as trivial (ES = 0.01–0.09), low to moderate (0.10–0.29), moderate to substantial (0.30–0.49), substantial to very strong (0.50–0.69), very strong (0.70–0.89), and almost perfect (0.90–0.99).

Researchers display the results of meta-analysis of the included individual studies in a forest plot graph. A forest plot shows the variation between the studies and an estimate of the overall result of all the studies together. This is usually accompanied by a table listing references (author and date) of the studies included in the meta-analysis and the statistical results (Centre for Evidence-Based Intervention, n.d.).

> **Example: Meta-Analysis**
>
> Meserve and colleagues (2021) conducted a meta-analysis of randomized controlled trials, cohort studies, and case series to evaluate the risks and outcomes of adverse events in patients with preexisting inflammatory bowel diseases treated with immune checkpoint inhibitors. They identified 12 studies reporting the impact of immune checkpoint inhibitors in 193 patients with inflammatory bowel disease and calculated pooled rates (with 95% confidence intervals [CI]) and examined risk factors associated with adverse outcomes through qualitative synthesis of individual studies. Approximately 40% of patients with preexisting inflammatory bowel diseases experienced relapse with immune checkpoint inhibitors, with most relapsing patients requiring corticosteroids and one-third requiring biologics.

Systematic Review With Meta-Synthesis

Meta-synthesis is the qualitative counterpart to meta-analysis. It involves interpreting data from multiple sources to produce a high-level narrative rather than aggregating data or producing a summary statistic. Meta-synthesis supports developing a broader interpretation than can be gained from a single primary qualitative study by combing the results from several qualitative studies to arrive at a deeper understanding of the phenomenon under review (Polit & Beck, 2017).

> **Example: Meta-Synthesis**
>
> Danielis et al. (2020) conducted a meta-synthesis and meta-summary to understand the physical and emotional experiences of adult intensive care unit (ICU) patients who receive mechanical ventilation. They searched four electronic databases and used the Critical Appraisal Skills Programme checklist to evaluate articles on their methodological quality. Nine studies met the criteria. The researchers identified twenty-four codes across eleven categories that indicated a need for improvements in clinical care, education, and policy to address this populations' feelings associated with fear, inability to communicate, and "feeling supervised."

Sources of Systematic Reviews

The Institute of Medicine (2011) appointed an expert committee to establish methodological standards for developing and reporting of all types of systematic reviews. The Agency for Healthcare Research and Quality (AHRQ), the lead federal agency charged with improving America's healthcare system's safety and quality, awards five-year contracts to North American institutions to serve as Evidence-Based Practice Centers (EPCs). EPCs review scientific literature on clinical, behavioral, organizational, and financial topics to produce evidence reports and technology assessments (AHRQ, 2016). Additionally, EPCs conduct research on systematic review methodology.

Research designs for conducting summaries of multiple studies include systematic reviews, meta-analysis (quantitative data), meta-synthesis (qualitative), and mixed methods (both quantitative and qualitative data). See Table 6.5 for national and international organizations that generate summaries of multiple studies.

Table 6.5 Organizations That Generate Summaries of Multiple Studies

Organization	Description
Agency for Healthcare Research and Quality (AHRQ)	The AHRQ Effective Health Care Program has several tools and resources for consumers, clinicians, policymakers, and others to make informed healthcare decisions.
AHRQ Methods Guide for Effectiveness and Comparative Effectiveness Reviews	
The Campbell Collaboration	The Campbell Collaboration is an international research network that produces systematic reviews of the effects of social interventions.
Centre for Reviews and Dissemination (CRD)	The Centre for Reviews and Dissemination provides research-based information about the effects of health and social care interventions and provides guidance on the undertaking of systematic reviews.

Cochrane Collaboration	The Cochrane Collaboration is an international organization that helps prepare and maintain the results of systematic reviews of healthcare interventions. Systematic reviews are disseminated through the online Cochrane Library, which is accessible through this guide and under databases on the NIH Library website.
JBI	JBI (formerly the Joanna Briggs Institute) is an international not-for-profit research and development Centre within the Faculty of Health Sciences and Medical at the University of Adelaide, South Australia that produces systematic reviews. JBI also provides comprehensive systematic review training.

Mixed-Methods Studies

As with quantitative and qualitative approaches, there are different designs within mixed methods (see Table 6.6). The most common mixed-method designs are convergent parallel, explanatory sequential, exploratory sequential, and multiphasic (Creswell & Plano Clark, 2018).

Table 6.6 Mixed-Methods Design, Procedure, and Use

Design	Procedure	Use
Convergent parallel	Concurrently conducts quantitative and qualitative elements in the same phase of the research process, weighs the methods equally, analyzes the two components independently, and interprets the results together	Validate quantitative scales and form a more complete understanding of a research topic
Explanatory sequential	Sequential design with quantitative data collected in the initial phase, followed by qualitative data	Used when quantitative findings are explained and interpreted with the assistance of qualitative data

continues

Table 6.6   Mixed-Methods Design, Procedure, and Use (cont.)

Design	Procedure	Use
Exploratory sequential designs	Sequential design with qualitative data collected in the initial phase, followed by quantitative data	Qualitative results need to be tested or generalized or for theory development or instrument development
Multiphasic	Combines the concurrent or sequential collection of quantitative and qualitative data sets over multiple phases of a study	Useful in comprehensive program evaluations by addressing a set of incremental research questions focused on a central objective

Determining the Level of Research Evidence

The JHEBP model encompasses quantitative and qualitative studies, primary studies, and summaries of multiple studies within three levels of evidence. The level of research evidence (true experimental, quasi-experimental, nonexperimental) is an objective determination based on the study design meeting the scientific evidence design requirements—manipulation of a variable in the form of an intervention, a control group, and random assignment to the intervention or control group. Table 6.7 identifies the type of research studies in each of the three levels of scientific evidence. The Research Appraisal Tool (Appendix E) provides specific criteria and decision points for determining the level of research evidence.

Table 6.7 Rating the Level of Research Evidence

Level	Type of Evidence
I	A true experimental study, randomized controlled trial (RCT), or systematic review of RCTs, with or without meta-analysis
II	A quasi-experimental study or systematic review of a combination of RCTs and quasi-experimental studies, or quasi-experimental studies only, with or without meta-analysis

| III | A quantitative nonexperimental study; systematic review of a combination of RCTs, quasi-experimental, and nonexperimental studies, or nonexperimental studies only; or qualitative study or systematic review of qualitative studies, with or without a meta-synthesis |

Appraising the Quality of Research Evidence

After the EBP team has determined the level of research evidence, the team evaluates the quality of the evidence with the corresponding expectations of the chosen study design. Individual elements to be evaluated for each piece of evidence will depend on the type of evidence but can include the quality (validity and reliability) of the researchers' measurements, statistical findings, and quality of reporting.

Quality of Measurement

Findings of research studies are only as good as the tools used to gather the data. Understanding and evaluating the psychometric properties of a given instrument, such as validity and reliability, allow for an in-depth understanding of the quality of the measurement.

Validity

Validity refers to the credibility of the research—the extent to which the research measures what it claims to measure. The validity of research is important because if the study does not measure what it intended, the results will not effectively answer the aim of the research. There are several ways to ensure validity, including expert review, Delphi studies, comparison with established tools, factor analysis, item response theory, and correlation tests (expressed as a correlation coefficient). There are two aspects of validity to measure: internal and external.

Internal validity is the degree to which observed changes in the dependent variable are due to the experimental treatment or intervention rather than other possible causes. An EBP team should question whether there are competing explanations for the observed results. Measures of internal validity include *content validity* (the extent to which a multi-item tool reflects the full extent of the construct being measured), *construct validity* (how well an instrument truly measures the concept of interest), and *cross-cultural validity* (how well a translated or culturally adapted tool performs relative to the original instrument) (Polit & Beck, 2017).

External validity refers to the likelihood that conclusions about research findings are generalizable to other settings or samples. Errors of measurement that affect validity can be systematic or constant. External validity is a significant concern with EBP when translating research into the real world or from one population/setting to another. An EBP team should question the extent to which study conclusions may reasonably hold true for their particular patient population and setting. Do the investigators state the participation rates of subjects and settings? Do they explain the intended target audience for the intervention or treatment? How representative is the sample of the population of interest? Ensuring the study participants' representativeness and replicating the study in multiple sites that differ in dimensions such as size, setting, and staff skill set improve external validity.

Experimental studies are high in internal validity because they are structured and control for extraneous variables. However, because of this, the generalizability of the results (external validity) may be limited. In contrast, nonexperimental and observational studies may be high in generalizability because the studies are conducted in real-world settings but are low on internal validity because of the inability to control variables that may affect the results.

Bias plays a large role in the potential validity of research findings. In the context of research, bias can present as preferences for, or prejudices against, particular groups or concepts. Bias occurs in all research, at any stage, and is difficult to eliminate. Table 6.8 outlines the types of bias.

Table 6.8 Types of Research Bias, Descriptions, and Mitigation Techniques

Type of Bias	Description	Mitigation Techniques
Investigator bias	Researcher unknowingly influences study participants' responses. Participants may pick up on subtle details in survey questions or their interaction with a study team member and conclude that they should respond a certain way.	Standardize all interactions with participants through interview scripts, and blind the collection or analysis of data.
Hawthorne effect	Changes in participants' behavior because they are aware that others are observing them.	Evaluate the value of direct observation over other data collection methods.
Attrition bias	Loss of participants during a study and the effect on representativeness within the sample. This can affect results, as the participants who remain in a study may collectively possess different characteristics than those who drop out.	Limit burden on participants while maximizing opportunities for engagement, communicating effectively and efficiently.
Selection bias	Nonrandom selection of samples. This can include allowing participants to self-select treatment options or assigning participants based upon specific demographics.	When possible, use a random sample. If not possible, apply rigorous inclusion and exclusion criteria to ensure recruitment occurs within the appropriate population while avoiding confounding factors. Use a large sample size.

Reliability

Reliability refers to the consistency of a set of measurements or an instrument used to measure a construct. For example, a patient scale is off by 5 pounds. When weighing the patient three times, the scale reads 137 every time (reliability). However, the weight is not the patient's true weight because the scale is not recording correctly (validity). Reliability refers, in essence, to the repeatability of a measurement. Errors of measurement that affect reliability are random. For example, variation in measurements may exist when nurses use patient care equipment such as blood pressure cuffs or glucometers. Table 6.9 displays three methods used to measure reliability: internal consistency reliability, test-retest reliability, and interrater reliability.

Evaluating Statistical Findings

Most research evidence will include reports of descriptive and analytic statistics of their study findings. The EBP team must understand the general concepts of common data analysis techniques to evaluate the meaning of study findings.

Measures of Central Tendency

Measures of *central tendency* (mean, median, and mode) are summary statistics that describe a set of data by identifying the central position within that set of data. The most well-known measure of central tendency is the *mean* (or average), which is used with both discrete data (based on counts) and continuous data (infinite number of values divided along a specified continuum) (Polit & Beck, 2017). Although a good measure of central tendency in normal distributions, the mean is misleading in skewed (asymmetric) distributions and extreme scores. The *median*, the number that lies at the midpoint of a distribution of values, is less sensitive to extreme scores and is therefore of greater use in skewed distributions. The *mode* is the most frequently occurring value and is the only measure of central tendency used with categorical data (data divided into groups). *Standard deviation* is the measure of scattering of a set of data from its mean. The more spread out a data distribution is, the greater its standard deviation. Standard deviation cannot be negative. A standard deviation close to 0 indicates that the data points tend to be close to the mean.

Table 6.9 Reliability Definitions and Statistical Techniques

Type of Reliability	Definition	Statistical Techniques
Internal consistency	Whether a set of items in an instrument or subscale that propose to measure the same construct produce similar scores.	Cronbach's alpha (α) is a coefficient of reliability (or consistency). Cronbach alpha values of 0.7 or higher indicate acceptable internal consistency.
Test-retest reliability	Degree to which scores are consistent over time. Indicates score variation that occurs from test session to test session that is a result of errors of measurement.	Pearson's r correlation coefficient (expresses the strength of a relationship between variables ranging from −1.00, a perfect negative correlation, to +1.00, a perfect positive relationship). Scatter plot data.
Interrater reliability	Extent to which two or more raters, observers, coders, examiners agree.	Techniques depend on what is actually being measured: ■ Correlational coefficients are used to measure consistency between raters ■ Percent agreement measures agreement between raters
Interrater reliability (cont.)		And the type of data: ■ Nominal data: also called categorical data; variables that have no value (e.g., gender, employment status) ■ Ordinal data: categorical data where order is important (e.g., Likert scale measuring level of happiness) ■ Interval data: numeric scales with a specified order and the exact differences between the values (e.g., blood pressure reading)

Measures of Statistical Significance

Statistical significance indicates whether findings reflect an actual association or difference between the variables/groups or are due to chance alone. The classic measure of statistical significance, the *p-value,* is a probability range from 0 to 1. The smaller the p-value (the closer it is to 0), the more likely the result is statistically significant. Factors that affect the p-value include sample size and the magnitude of the difference between groups (effect size) (Thiese et al., 2016).

For example, if the sample size is large enough, the results are more likely to show a significant p-value, even if the effect size is small or clinically insignificant, but there is a true difference in the groups. In healthcare literature, the p-value for determining statistical significance is generally set at $p < 0.05$.

Though p-values indicate statistical significance (i.e., the results are not due to chance), healthcare research results are increasingly reporting effect sizes and confidence intervals to more fully interpret results and guide decisions for translation. *Effective sizes* are the amount of difference between two groups. A positive effect size indicates a positive relationship—as one variable increases, the second variable increases. A negative effect size signifies a negative relationship, where as one variable increases or decreases, the second variable moves in the opposite direction. *Confidence intervals* (CI) are a measure of precision and are expressed as a range of values (upper limit and lower limit) where a given measure actually lies based on a predetermined probability. The standard 95% CI means an investigator can be 95% confident that the actual values in a given population fall within the upper and lower limits of the range of values.

Quality of Reporting

Regardless of the quality of the conduct of a research investigation, the implications of that study cannot be adequately determined if the researchers do not provide a complete and detailed report. The Enhancing the QUAlity and Transparency Of health Research (EQUATOR) network (https://www.equator-network.org) is a repository of reporting guidelines organized by study type. These guidelines provide a road map for the required steps to conduct and report out a robust study. While ideally researchers are using standard reporting guidelines, the degree to which journals demand adherence to these standards varies. Regardless of the type of study, classic elements of published research include *title, abstract, introduction, methods, results, discussion,* and *conclusion* (Lunsford & Lunsford, 1996).

Title

Ideally, the title should be informative and help the reader understand the type of study being reported. A well-chosen title states what the author did, to whom it was done, and how it was done. Consider the title "Improving transitions in care for children with complex and medically fragile needs: a mixed-methods study" (Curran et al., 2020). The reader is immediately apprised of what was done (improve transitions in care), to whom it was done (children with complex and medically fragile needs), and how it was done (a mixed-methods study).

Abstract

The abstract is often located after the title and author section and graphically set apart by the use of a box, shading, or italics. The abstract is a brief description of the problem, methods, and findings of the study (Polit & Beck, 2017).

Introduction

The introduction contains the background and a problem statement that tells why the investigators have chosen to conduct the study. The best way to present the background is by reporting on current literature, and the author should identify the knowledge gap between what is known and what the study seeks to find out (or answer). A clear, direct statement of purpose and a statement of expected results or hypotheses should be included.

Methods

This section describes how a study is conducted (study procedures) in sufficient detail so that readers can replicate the study, including the study design, population with inclusion and exclusion criteria, recruitment, consent, a description of the intervention, and how data was collected and analyzed. If instrumentation was used, the methods section should include the validity and reliability of the tools. Authors should also include an acknowledgment of ethical review for research studies involving human subjects. The methods should read similar to a manual of the study design.

Results

Study results list the findings of the data analysis and should not contain commentary. Give particular attention to figures and tables, which are the heart of most papers. Look to see whether results report statistical versus clinical significance, and look up unfamiliar terminology, symbols, or logic.

Discussion

The discussion should align with the introduction and results and state the implications of the findings. This section explores the research findings and meaning given to the results, including how they compare to similar studies. Authors should also identify the study's main weaknesses or limitations and identify the actions taken to minimize them.

Conclusion

The conclusion should contain a brief restatement of the experimental results and implications of the study (Hall, 2012). If the conclusion does not have a separate header, it usually falls at the end of the discussion section.

The Overall Report

The parts of the research article should be highly interconnected (but not overlap). The researcher needs to ensure that any hypotheses flow directly from the review of literature, and results support arguments or interpretations presented in the discussion and conclusion sections.

Determining the Quality of Evidence

Rating the quality of research evidence includes considerations of factors such as sample size (power of study to detect true differences), extent to which you can generalize the findings from a sample to an entire population, and validity (indicates findings truly represent the phenomenon you are claiming to measure). In contrast to the objective approach to determining the level, grading the quality of evidence is subjective and requires critical thinking by the EBP team to make a determination (see Table 6.10).

Table 6.10 Quality Rating for Research Evidence

Grade	Research Evidence
A: High	Consistent, generalizable results; sufficient sample size for study design; adequate control; definitive conclusions; recommendations consistent with the study's findings and include thorough reference to scientific evidence
B: Good	Reasonably consistent results; sufficient sample size for the study design; some control; fairly definitive conclusions; recommendations reasonably consistent with the study's findings and include some reference to scientific evidence
C: Low	Little evidence with inconsistent results; insufficient sample size for the study design; conclusions cannot be drawn

Experimental Studies (Level I Evidence)

True experiments have a high degree of internal validity because manipulation and random assignment enables researchers to rule out most alternative explanations of results (Polit & Beck, 2017). Internal validity, however, decreases the generalizability of the results (external validity). To uncover potential threats to external validity, the EBP team may pose questions such as, "How confident are we that the study findings can transfer from the sample to the entire population? Are the study conditions as close as possible to real-world situations? Did subjects have inherent differences even before manipulation of the independent variable (selection bias)? Are participants responding in a certain way because they know the researcher is observing them (the Hawthorne effect)? Are there researcher behaviors or characteristics that may influence the subject's responses (investigator bias)? In multi-institutional studies, are there variations in how study coordinators at various sites managed the trial?

Subject mortality and different dropout rates between experimental and control groups may affect the adequacy of the sample size. Additional items the EBP team may want to assess related to reasons for dropout of subjects include whether the experimental treatment was painful or time-consuming and whether participants remaining in the study differ from those who dropped out. It is important to assess the nature of possible biases that may affect randomization. Assess for selection biases by comparing groups on pretest data (Polit & Beck, 2017). If there are no pretest measures, compare groups on demographic and disease variables such as age, health status, and ethnicity. If there are multiple data collection points, it is important to assess attrition biases by comparing those who did or did not complete the intervention. EBP teams should carefully analyze how the researchers address possible sources of bias.

Quasi-Experimental Studies (Level II Evidence)

As with true experimental studies, threats to generalizability (external validity) for quasi-experimental studies include maturation, testing, and instrumentation, with the additional threats of history and selection (Polit & Beck, 2017). The occurrence of external events during the study (threat of history) can affect a subject's response to the investigational intervention or treatment. Additionally, with nonrandomized groups, preexisting differences between the groups can affect the outcome. Questions the EBP team may pose to uncover potential threats to internal validity include, "Did some event occur during the study that may have influenced the results of the study? Are there processes occurring within subjects over the course of the study because of the passage of time (maturation) rather than from the experimental intervention? Could the pretest have influenced the subject's performance on the posttest? Were the measurement instruments and procedures the same for both points of data collection?"

In terms of external validity, threats associated with sampling design, such as patient selection and characteristics of nonrandomized patients, affect the general findings. External validity improves if the researcher uses random selection of subjects, even if random assignment to groups is not possible.

Nonexperimental and Qualitative Studies (Level III Evidence)

The evidence gained from well-designed nonexperimental and qualitative studies is the lowest level in the research hierarchy (Level III).

When looking for potential threats to external validity in quantitative nonexperimental studies, the EBP team can pose the questions described under experimental and quasi-experimental studies. In addition, the team may ask further questions such as, "Did the researcher attempt to control for extraneous variables with the use of careful subject-selection criteria? Did the researcher attempt to minimize the potential for socially acceptable responses by the subject? Did the study rely on documentation as the source of data? In methodological studies (developing, testing, and evaluating research instruments and methods), were the test subjects selected from the population for which the test will be used? Was the survey response rate high enough to generalize findings to the target population? For historical research studies, are the data authentic and genuine?"

Qualitative studies offer many challenges with respect to the question of validity. There are several suggested ways to determine validity, or rigor, in qualitative research. Four common approaches to establish rigor (Saumure & Given, 2012) are:

- **Transparency:** How clear the research process has been explained
- **Credibility:** The extent to which data are representative
- **Dependability:** Other researchers would draw the same or similar conclusions when looking at the data
- **Reflexivity:** How the researcher has reported how they were involved in the research and may have influenced the study results

Issues of rigor in qualitative research are complex, so the EBP team should appraise how well the researchers discuss how they determined validity for the particular study.

Systematic Reviews (Level I or II Evidence)

Teams should evaluate systematic reviews for the rigor and transparency they display in their search strategies, appraisal methods, and results. Systematic reviews should follow well-established reporting guidelines (Moher et al., 2009), in most cases, the Preferred Reporting Items for Systematic Reviews and Meta-Analyses (PRISMA). This includes a reproducible search strategy, a flow diagram of the literature screening, clear data extraction methodology and reporting, and methods used to evaluate the strength of the literature. Authors should ensure all conclusions are based on a critical evaluation of results.

Systematic Review With Meta-Analysis

The strength (level and quality) of the evidence on which recommendations are made within a meta-analytic study depends on the design and quality of studies included in the meta-analysis as well as the design of the meta-analysis itself. Factors to consider include sampling criteria of the primary studies included in the analysis, quality of the primary studies, and variation in outcomes between studies.

To determine the level, the EBP team looks at the types of research designs included in the meta-analysis. Meta-analyses containing only randomized controlled trials are Level I evidence. Some meta-analyses include data from quasi-experimental or nonexperimental studies, and the level of evidence would be at a level commensurate with the lowest level of research design included (e.g., if the meta-analysis included experimental and quasi-experimental studies, the meta-analysis would be Level II).

To determine the quality of the article, first the team should look at the strength of the individual studies included. For an EBP team to evaluate evidence obtained from a meta-analysis, the meta-analysis report must be detailed enough for the reader to understand the studies included. Second, the team should assess the quality of the meta-analysis itself. The discussion section should include an overall summary of the findings, the magnitude of the effect, the number of studies, and the combined sample size. The discussion should present the overall quality of the evidence and consistency of findings (Polit & Beck, 2017). The discussion should also include a recommendation for future research to improve the evidence base.

Systematic Review With Meta-Syntheses (Level III Evidence)

Evaluating and synthesizing qualitative research presents many challenges. It is not surprising that EBP teams may feel at a loss in assessing the quality of meta-synthesis. Approaching these reviews from a broad perspective enables the team to look for quality indicators that both quantitative and qualitative summative research techniques have in common.

The following should be noted in meta-synthesis reports: explicit search strategies, inclusion and exclusion criteria, methods used to determine study quality, methodological details for all included studies, and the conduct of the meta-synthesis itself. Similar to other summative approaches, a

> *meta-synthesis should be undertaken by a team of experts since the application of multiple perspectives to the processes of study appraisal, coding, charting, mapping, and interpretation may result in additional insights, and thus in a more complete interpretation of the subject of the review* (Jones, 2004, p. 277).

EBP teams need to keep in mind that judgments related to study strengths and weaknesses as well as to the suitability of recommendations for the target population are both context-specific and dependent on the question asked. Some conditions or circumstances, such as clinical setting or time of day, are relevant to determining a particular recommended intervention's applicability.

A Practical Tool for Appraising Research Evidence

The Research Evidence Appraisal Tool (see Appendix E) gauges the level and quality of research evidence. The tool contains questions to guide the team in determining the level and the quality of evidence of the primary studies included in the review. Strength (level and quality) is higher with evidence from at least one well-designed (quality), randomized controlled trial (RCT) (Level I) than from at least one well-designed quasi-experimental (Level II), nonexperimental and qualitative (Level III) study. After determining the level, the tool contains additional questions specific to the study methods and execution to determine the quality of the research.

Recommendations for Interprofessional Leaders

Professional standards have long held that clinicians need to integrate the best available evidence, including research findings, into practice and practice decisions. This is the primary way to use new knowledge gained from research. Research articles can be intimidating to novice and expert nurses alike. Leaders can best support EBP by providing clinicians with the resources to appraise research evidence. It is highly recommended that they make available research texts, mentors, or experts to assist teams to become competent consumers of research. Only through continuous learning can clinicians gain the confidence needed to incorporate evidence gleaned from research into individual patients' day-to-day care.

Summary

This chapter arms EBP teams with practical information to guide the appraisal of research evidence, a task that is often difficult for nonresearchers. It presents an overview of the various types of research evidence, including attention to individual research studies and summaries of multiple research studies. Strategies and tips for reading research reports guide team members on how to appraise the strength (level and quality) of research evidence.

References

Agency for Healthcare Research and Quality. (2016). *EPC evidence-based reports*. Content last reviewed March, 2021. http://www.ahrq.gov/research/findings/evidence-based-reports/index.html

Aromataris, E., & Munn, Z. (2020). JBI systematic reviews. In E. Aromataris & Z. Munn (Eds.), *JBI manual for evidence synthesis* (Chapter 1). JBI. https://synthesismanual.jbi.global

Awoke, M. S., Baptiste, D. L., Davidson, P., Roberts, A., & Dennison-Himmelfarb, C. (2019). A quasi-experimental study examining a nurse-led education program to improve knowledge, self-care, and reduce readmission for individuals with heart failure. *Contemporary Nurse*, *55*(1), 15–26. https://doi.org/10.1080/10376178.2019.1568198

Centre for Evidence-Based Intervention. (n.d.). https://www.spi.ox.ac.uk/what-is-good-evidence#/

Cohen, J. (1988). *Statistical power analysis for the behavioral sciences*. Academic Press.

Creswell, J. W., & Creswell, J. D. (2018). *Research design: Qualitative, quantitative, and mixed methods approaches* (5th ed.). SAGE Publishing.

Creswell, J. W., & Plano Clarke, V. L. (2018). *Designing and conducting mixed methods research* (3rd ed.). SAGE Publishing.

Curran, J. A., Breneol, S., & Vine, J. (2020). Improving transitions in care for children with complex and medically fragile needs: A mixed methods study. *BMC Pediatrics*, *20*(1), 1–14. https://doi.org/10.1186/s12887-020-02117-6

Daniclis, M., Povoli, A., Mattiussi, E., & Palese, A. (2020). Understanding patients' experiences of being mechanically ventilated in the Intensive Care Unit: Findings from a meta synthesis and meta summary. *Journal of Clinical Nursing*, *29*(13–14), 2107–2124. https://doi.org/10.1111/jocn.15259

Grant, M. J., & Booth, A. (2009). A typology of reviews: An analysis of 14 review types and associated methodologies. *Health Information and Libraries Journal*, *26*(2), 91–108. https://doi.org/10.1111/j.1471-1842.2009.00848.x

Hall, G. M. (Ed.). (2012). *How to write a paper*. John Wiley & Sons.

Institute of Medicine. (2011). *Finding what works in health care standards for systematic reviews*. National Academy of Sciences.

Jones, M. L. (2004). Application of systematic review methods to qualitative research: Practical issues. *Journal of Advanced Nursing*, *48*(3), 271–278. https://doi.org/10.1111/j.1365-2648.2004.03196.x

Lunsford, T. R., & Lunsford, B. R. (1996). Research forum: How to critically read a journal research article. *Journal of Prosthetics and Orthotics*, *8*(1), 24–31.

Meserve, J., Facciorusso, A., Holmer, A. K., Annese, V., Sanborn, W., & Singh, S. (2021). Systematic review with meta-analysis: Safety and tolerability of immune checkpoint inhibitors in patients with pre-existing inflammatory bowel diseases. *Alimentary Pharmacology & Therapeutics*, *53*(3), 374–382.

Moher, D., Liberati, A., Tetzlaff, J., & Altman, D., G. for the PRISMA Group. (2009). Preferred reporting items for systematic reviews and meta-analyses: The PRISMA statement. *BMJ*, *339*, b2535. https://doi.org/10.1136/bmj.b2535

Polit, D. F., & Beck, C. T. (2017). *Nursing research: Generating and assessing evidence for nursing practice* (10th ed.). Lippincott Williams & Wilkens.

Rahmani, B., Aghebati, N., Esmaily, H., & Florczak, K. L. (2020). Nurse-led care program with patients with heart failure using Johnson's Behavioral System Model: A randomized controlled trial. *Nursing Science Quarterly, 33*(3), 204–214. https://doi.org/10.1177/0894318420932102

Saumure, K., & Given, L. M. (2012). Rigor in qualitative research. In L. M. Given (Ed.). *The SAGE encyclopedia of qualitative research methods,* 795–796. SAGE Publishing.

Thiese, M. S., Ronna, B., & Ott, U. (2016). P value interpretations and considerations. *Journal of Thoracic Disease,* (9), E928–E931. https://doi.org/10.21037/jtd.2016.08.16

Evidence Appraisal: Nonresearch

A distinguishing feature and strength of EBP is the inclusion of multiple evidence sources. In addition to research evidence, clinicians can draw from a range of nonresearch evidence to inform their practice. Such evidence includes personal, aesthetic, and ethical ways of knowing (Carper, 1978)—for example, the expertise, experience, and values of individual practitioners, patients, and patients' families. In this chapter, nonresearch evidence is divided into summaries of evidence (clinical practice guidelines, consensus or position statements, literature reviews); organizational experience (quality improvement and financial data); expert opinion (commentary or opinion, case reports); community standards; clinician experience; and consumer preferences. This chapter:

- Describes types of nonresearch evidence
- Explains strategies for evaluating such evidence
- Recommends approaches for building clinicians' capacity to appraise nonresearch evidence to inform their practice

Summaries of Research Evidence

Summaries of research evidence such as clinical practice guidelines, consensus or position statements, integrative reviews, and literature reviews are excellent sources of information relevant to practice questions. These forms of evidence review and summarize all research, not just experimental studies. They are not themselves classified as research evidence because they are often not comprehensive and may not include an appraisal of study quality.

Clinical Practice Guidelines and Consensus/Position Statements (Level IV Evidence)

Clinical practice guidelines (CPGs), as defined by the Institute of Medicine (IOM) in 2011, are statements that include recommendations intended to optimize patient care that are informed by a systematic review of evidence and an assessment of the benefits and harms of alternative care (IOM, 2011). CPGs are tools designed to provide structured guidance about evidence-based care, which can decrease variability in healthcare delivery, improving patient outcomes (Abrahamson et al., 2012).

A key aspect of developing a valuable and trusted guideline is creation by a guideline development group representing stakeholders with a wide range of expertise, such as clinician generalists and specialists, content experts, methodologists, public health specialists, economists, patients, and advocates (Sniderman & Furberg, 2009; Tunkel & Jones, 2015). The expert panelists should provide full disclosure and accounting of how they addressed intellectual and financial conflicts that could influence the guidelines (Joshi et al., 2019). The guideline development group should use a rigorous process for assembling, evaluating, and summarizing the published evidence to develop the CPG recommendations (Ransohoff et al., 2013). The strength of the recommendations should be graded to provide transparency about the certainty of the data and values applied in the process (Dahm et al., 2009). The Grading of Recommendations, Assessment, Development and Evaluations (GRADE) strategy is a commonly used system to assess the strength of CPG recommendations (weak or strong), as well as the quality of evidence (high, moderate, low/very low) they are based on (Neumann et al., 2016). For example, a 1A recommendation is one that is strong and is based on high-quality evidence. This system has been widely adopted by organizations such as the World Health Organization (WHO), as well as groups such as the American College of Chest Physicians (CHEST). Use of consistent grading systems can align evidence synthesis methods and result in more explicit and easier-to-understand recommendations for the end user (Diekemper et al., 2018).

Consensus or position statements (CSs) may be developed instead of a CPG when the available evidence is insufficient due to lack of high-quality evidence or conflicting evidence, or scenarios where assessing benefits and risks of an intervention are challenging (Joshi et al., 2019). *Consensus statements* (CSs) are broad statements of best practice based on consensus opinion of the convened expert panel and possibly small bodies of evidence; are most often meant to guide members of a professional organization in decision-making; and may not provide specific algorithms for practice (Lopez-Olivo et al., 2008).

Hundreds of different groups have developed several thousand different CPGs and CSs (Ransohoff et al., 2013). It has been noted that the methodological quality of CPGs varies considerably by developing organizations, creating clinician concerns over the use of guidelines and potential impact on patients (Dahm et al., 2009). Formal methods have been developed to assess the quality of CPGs. A group of researchers from 13 countries, Appraisal of Guidelines Research and Evaluation (AGREE) Collaboration, developed a guideline appraisal instrument with documented reliability and validity. It has been shown that high-quality guidelines were more often produced by government-supported organizations or a structured, coordinated program (Fervers et al., 2005). The AGREE instrument, revised in 2013, now has 23 items and is organized into six domains (The AGREE Research Trust, 2013; Brouwers et al., 2010):

- Scope and purpose
- Stakeholder involvement
- Rigor of development
- Clarity of presentation
- Applicability
- Editorial independence

Despite the availability of the AGREE tool and others like it, the quality of guidelines still vary greatly in terms of how they are developed and how the results are reported (Kuehn, 2011). A recent evaluation of more than 600 CPGs found that while quality of the CPGs has increased over time, the quality scores assessed by the tool have remained moderate to low (Alonso-Coello, 2010). In response to concern about CPG quality, an IOM committee was commissioned to study the CPG development process. The committee (IOM, 2011) developed a comprehensive set of criteria outlining "standards for trustworthiness" for clinical practice guidelines development (see Table 7.1).

Table 7.1 Clinical Practice Guideline (CPG) Standards and Description

Standard	Description
Establish transparency	Funding and development process should be publicly available.
Disclose conflict(s) of interest (COI)	Individuals who create guidelines and panel chairs should be free from conflicts of interest (COI). Funders are excluded from CPG development. All COIs of each guideline development group member should be disclosed.
Balance membership of guideline development group	Guideline developers should include multiple disciplines, patients, patient advocates, or patient consumer organizations.
Use systematic reviews	CPG developers should use systematic reviews that meet IOM's Standards for Systematic Reviews of Comparative Effectiveness Research.
Rate strength of evidence and recommendations	Rating has specified criteria rating the level of evidence and strength of recommendations.
Articulate recommendations	Recommendations should follow a standard format and be worded so that compliance can be evaluated.

External review	External reviews should represent all relevant stakeholders. A draft of the CPG should be available to the public at the external review stage or directly afterward.
Update guidelines	CPGs should be updated when new evidence suggests the need, and the CPG publication date, date of systematic evidence review, and proposed date for future review should be documented.

For more than 20 years, the National Guideline Clearinghouse (NGC), an initiative of the Agency for Healthcare Research and Quality (AHRQ), US Department of Health and Human Services, was a source of high-quality guidelines and rigorous standards. This initiative was ended due to lack of funding in 2018. At that time, the Emergency Care Research Institute (ECRI), a non-profit, independent organization servicing the healthcare industry, committed to continuing the legacy of the NGC by creating the ECRI Guidelines Trust. The trust houses hundreds of guidelines on its website, which is free to access (https://guidelines.ecri.org). ECRI summarizes guidelines in snapshots and briefs and appraises them against the Institute of Medicine (IOM) Standards for Trustworthy Guidelines by using TRUST (Transparency and Rigor Using Standards of Trustworthiness) scorecards (ECRI, 2020). This source can be useful to EBP teams needing guidelines for evidence appraisals.

Literature Reviews (Level V Evidence)

Literature review is a broad term that refers to a summary or synthesis of published literature without systematic appraisal of evidence quality or strength. The terminology of literature reviews has evolved into many different types, with different search processes and degrees of rigor (Peters et al., 2015; Snyder, 2019; Toronto et al., 2018). Traditional literature reviews are not confined to scientific literature; a review may include nonscientific literature such as theoretical papers, reports of organizational experience, and opinions of experts. Such reviews possess some of the desired attributes of a systematic review, but not the same standardized approach, appraisal, and critical review of the studies. Literature review types also vary in completeness and often lack the intent of including all available evidence on a topic (Grant & Booth, 2009). Qualities of different types of literature reviews and their product are outlined in Table 7.2.

Specific challenges may arise in conducting or reading a literature review. One challenge is that not all the articles returned in the search answer the specific questions being posed. When conducting a literature search, attention to the details of the search parameters—such as the Boolean operators or using the correct Medical Subject Headings (MeSH)—may provide a more comprehensive search, as described in Chapter 5. Shortcomings of available literature should be described in the limitations section. If only some of the articles answer the questions posed while reading a literature review, the reader must interpret the findings more carefully and may need to identify additional literature reviews that answer the remaining questions. Another common problem in literature reviews is double counting of study results, which may influence the results of the literature review. Double counting can take many forms, including simple double counting of the same study in two included meta-analyses, double counting of control arms between two interventions, imputing data missing from included studies, incomplete reporting of data in the included studies, and others (Senn, 2009). Recommendations to reduce the incidence of double counting include vigilance about double counting, making results verifiable, describing analysis in detail, judging the process not the author in review, and creating a culture of correction (Senn, 2009).

Integrative Reviews (Level V Evidence)

An *integrative review* is more rigorous than a literature review but lacks the methodical rigor of a systematic review with or without meta-analysis. It summarizes evidence that is a combination of research and theoretical literature and draws from manuscripts using varied methodologies (e.g., experimental, non-experimental, qualitative). The purpose of an integrative review varies widely compared to a systematic review; these purposes include summarizing evidence, reviewing theories, defining concepts, and other purposes. Well-defined and clearly presented search and selection strategies are critical. Because diverse methodologies may be combined in an integrative review, quality evaluation or further analysis of data is complex. Unlike the literature review, however, an integrative review analyzes, compares themes, and notes gaps in the selected literature (Whittemore & Knafl, 2005).

Table 7.2   Types of Literature Review

Type	Characteristics	Result
Literature review	An examination of current literature on a topic of interest. The purpose is to create context for an inquiry topic. Lack a standardized approach for critical appraisal and review. Often includes diverse types of evidence.	Summation or identification of gaps
Critical review	Extensive literature research from diverse sources, but lacks systematicity. Involves analysis and synthesis of results, but focuses on conceptual contribution of the papers, not their quality.	A hypothesis or model
Rapid review	Time-sensitive assessment of current knowledge of practice or policy issue, using systematic review methods. Time savings by focus on narrow scope, using less comprehensive search, extracting only key variables, or performing less rigorous quality appraisal. Increased risk of bias due to limited time frame of literature or quality analysis.	Timely review of current event or policy
Qualitative systematic review	Method to compare or integrate finding from qualitative studies, to identify themes or constructs in or across qualitative studies. Useful when knowledge of preferences and attitudes are needed. Standards for performing this type of review are in early stages, so rigor may vary.	New theory, narrative, or wider understanding
Scoping review	Determines nature and extent of available research evidence, or maps a body of literature to identify boundaries of research evidence. Limitations in rigor and duration increase risk of bias. Limited quality assessment.	Identify gaps in research, clarify key concepts, report on types of evidence

continues

Table 7.2   Types of Literature Review (cont.)

Type	Characteristics	Result
State-of-the-art review	A type of literature review that addresses more current matters than literature review. Review may encompass a recent period, so could miss important earlier works.	New perspectives on an issue or an area in need of research
Systematized review	Includes some, but not all, elements of systematic review. Search strategies are typically more systematic than other literature reviews, but synthesis and quality assessment are often lacking.	Form a basis for further complete systematic review or dissertation

Interpreting Evidence From Summaries of Research Evidence

Evaluating the quality of research that composes a body of evidence, for the purpose of developing CPGs, CSs, or performing a literature review, can be difficult. In 1996, editors of leading medical journals and researchers developed an initial set of guidelines for reporting results of randomized controlled clinical trials, which resulted in the CONsolidated Standards of Reporting Trials (CONSORT) Statement (Altman & Simera, 2016). Following revisions to the initial CONSORT flowchart and checklist, the Enhancing the QUality and Transparency Of health Research (EQUATOR) program was started in 2006. Since then, the EQUATOR Network has developed reporting guidelines for many different types of research, including observational studies, systematic reviews, case reports, qualitative studies, quality improvement reports, and clinical practice guidelines (EQUATOR Network, n.d.). These guidelines have made it easier to assess the quality of research reports. However, no similar guidelines exist for assessing the quality of nonsystematic literature reviews or integrative reviews.

The Institute of Medicine (IOM, now the National Academy of Medicine) publication *Clinical Practice Guidelines We Can Trust* established standards for CPGs to be "informed by a systematic review of evidence and an assessment of the benefits and harms of alternative care options" (IOM, 2011, p. 4).

This standardization reduced the number of guidelines available in the National Guideline Clearinghouse by nearly 50% (Shekelle, 2018). However, the number of guidelines then rapidly increased, often covering the same topic but developed by different organizations, which led to redundancy if the guidelines were similar, or uncertainty when guidelines differed between organizations (Shekelle, 2018). The National Guideline Clearinghouse free access was eliminated in 2018 and replaced with the ECRI Trust. Limited evidence or conflicting recommendations require that the healthcare professional utilize critical thinking and clinical judgment when making clinical recommendations to healthcare consumers. Guidelines are intended to apply to the majority of clinical situations, but the unique needs of specific patients may also require the use of clinician judgment.

Clinical practice guideline development, as well as utilization, also needs to consider *health inequity*, avoidable differences in health that are rooted in lack of fairness or injustice (Welch et al., 2017). Characteristics to consider include the acronym PROGRESS-Plus: place of residence, race/ethnicity/culture/language, occupation, gender, religion, education, socioeconomic status, social capital; plus others including age, disability, sexual orientation, time-dependent situations, and relationships. Barriers to care associated with these characteristics are related to access to care/systems issues or provider/patient behaviors, attitudes, and conscious or unconscious biases (Welch et al., 2017). Some of these characteristics merit their own guideline; for example, a guideline related to asthma care for adults may not be applicable to the care of children with asthma.

Because guidelines are developed from systematic reviews, EBP teams should consider that although groups of experts create these guidelines, which frequently carry a professional society's seal of approval, the opinions of guideline developers that convert data to recommendations require subjective judgments that, in turn, leave room for error and bias (Mims, 2015). Actual and potential conflicts of interest are increasingly common within organizations and experts who create CPGs. Conflicts of interest may encompass more than industry relationships; for example, a guideline that recommends increased medical testing and visits may also serve the interests of clinicians, if they are the sole or predominate members of the guideline development group (Shekelle, 2018). Conflicts of interest may also be the result of financial or leadership interests, job descriptions, personal research interests, or volunteer work for organizations, among others. The IOM panel recommended that, whenever possible, individuals who create the guidelines should be free from conflicts of interest; if that is not possible, however, those individuals with conflicts of interest should make up a minority of the panel and should not serve as chairs or cochairs (IOM, 2011). In addition, specialists who may benefit from implementation of the guideline should be in the minority.

Professional associations have purposes besides development of clinical practice guidelines, including publishing, providing education, and advocacy for public health as well as their members through political lobbying (Nissen, 2017). Relationships between medical industry, professional associations, and experts who develop guidelines must be carefully assessed for actual or potential conflicts of interest, and these conflicts must be transparently disclosed and managed. Relationships between healthcare providers and the medical industry are not inherently bad; these relationships foster innovation and development, allow a partnership of shared expertise, and keep clinicians informed of advances in treatment as well as their safe and effective use (Sullivan, 2018). However, there is potential for undue influence, so these relationships must be leveraged with transparency to prevent abuses (Sullivan, 2018).

Key elements to note when appraising Level IV evidence and rating evidence quality are identified in Table 7.3 and in the JHNEBP Nonresearch Evidence Appraisal Tool (see Appendix F). Not all these elements are required, but the attributes listed are some of the evaluative criteria.

Table 7.3 Desirable Attributes of Documents Used to Answer an EBP Question

Attribute	Question
Applicability to topic	Does the document address the particular practice question of interest (same intervention, same population, same setting)?
Comprehensiveness of search strategy	Do the authors identify search strategies beyond the typical databases, such as PubMed, PsycInfo, and CINAHL?
	Are published and unpublished works included?

Methodology	Do the authors clearly specify how inclusion and exclusion criteria were applied? Do the authors specify how data were analyzed?
Consistency of findings	Are the findings organized and synthesized in a clear and cohesive manner?
	Are tables organized, and do they summarize the findings in a concise manner?
Study quality assessment	Do the authors clearly describe how the review addresses study quality?
Limitations	Are methodological limitations disclosed? Has double counting been assessed?
Conclusions	Do the conclusions appear to be based on the evidence and capture the complexity of the topic?
Collective expertise	Was the review and synthesis done by an expert or group of experts?

Adapted from Conn (2004), Stetler et al. (1998), and Whittemore (2005).

Organizational Experience

Organizational experience often takes the form of quality improvement (QI) and economic or program evaluations. These sources of evidence can occur at any level in the organization and can be internal to an EBP team's organization or published reports from external organizations.

Quality Improvement Reports (Level V Evidence)

The Department of Health and Human Services defines *quality improvement* (QI) as "consisting of systematic and continuous actions that lead to measurable improvement in health care services and health status of targeted patient groups" (Connelly, 2018, p. 125). The term is used interchangeably with quality management, performance improvement, total quality management, and continuous quality improvement (Yoder-Wise, 2014). These terms refer to the application of improvement practices using tools and methods to examine workflows, processes, or systems within a specific organization with the aim of securing positive change in a particular service (Portela et al., 2015). QI uses process improvement techniques adapted from industry, such as Lean and Six Sigma frameworks, which employ incremental, cyclically implemented changes with Plan-Do-Study-Act (PDSA) cycles (Baker et al., 2014).

QI projects produce evidence of valuable results in local practice and may be published as quality improvement reports in journals (Carter et al., 2017). EBP teams are reminded that the focus of QI studies is to determine whether an intervention works to improve processes, and not necessarily for scientific advancement, which is the focus of health services research. Thus, lack of generalizability of results is a weakness, as is lack of structured explanations of mechanisms of change and low quality of reports (Portela et al., 2015).

During their review of nonresearch evidence, EBP team members should examine internal QI data relating to the practice question as well as QI initiatives based on similar questions published by peer institutions. As organizations become more mature in their QI efforts, they become more rigorous in the approach, the analysis of results, and the use of established measures as metrics (Newhouse et al., 2006). Organizations that may benefit from QI reports' published findings need to make decisions regarding implementation based on the characteristics of their organization.

As the number of quality improvement reports has grown, so has concern about the quality of reporting. In an effort to reduce uncertainty about what information should be included in scholarly reports of health improvement, the Standards for Quality Improvement Reporting Excellence (SQUIRE) were published in 2008 and revised in 2015 (http://www.squire-statement.org). The SQUIRE guidelines list and explain items that authors should consider including in a report of system-level work to improve healthcare (Ogrinc et al., 2015). Although evidence obtained from QI initiatives is not as strong as that obtained by scientific inquiry, the sharing of successful QI stories has the potential to identify future EBP questions, QI projects, and research studies external to the organization.

An example of a quality improvement project is a report from an emergency department (ED) and medical intensive care unit (MICU) on transfer time delays of critically ill patients from ED to MICU (Cohen et al., 2015). Using a clinical microsystems approach, the existing practice patterns were identified, and multiple causes that contributed to delays were determined. The Plan-Do-Study-Act model was applied in each intervention to reduce delays. The intervention reduced transfer time by 48% by improving coordination in multiple stages. This Level V evidence is from one institution that implemented a quality improvement project.

Economic Evaluation (Level V Evidence)

Economic measures in healthcare facilities provide data to assess the cost associated with practice changes. Cost savings assessments can be powerful information as the best practice is examined. In these partial economic evaluations, there is not a comparison of two or more alternatives but rather an explanation of the cost to achieve a particular outcome. Economic evaluations intended to evaluate quality improvement interventions in particular are mainly concerned with determining whether the investment in the intervention is justifiable (Portela et al., 2015).

Full economic evaluations apply analytic techniques to identify, measure, and compare the costs and outcomes of two or more alternative programs or interventions (Centers for Disease Control and Prevention [CDC], 2007). Costs in an economic analysis framework are the value of resources, either theoretical or monetary, associated with each treatment or intervention; the consequences are the health effects of the intervention (Gray & Wilkinson, 2016). A common economic evaluation of healthcare decision-making is a cost-effectiveness analysis, which compares costs of alternative interventions that produce a common health outcome in terms of clinical units (e.g., years of life). Although the results of such an analysis can provide justification for a program, empirical evidence can provide support for an increase in program funding or a switch from one program to another (CDC, 2007). Another type of full economic evaluation is cost benefit analysis. In this type of economic evaluation, both costs and benefits (or health effects) are expressed in monetary units (Gommersall et al., 2015). An EBP team can find reports of cost effectiveness and economic evaluations (Level V) in published data or internal organizational reports. One example is "The Value of Reducing Hospital-Acquired Pressure Ulcer Prevalence" (Spetz et al., 2013). This study assessed the cost savings associated with implementing nursing approaches to prevent hospital-acquired pressure ulcers (HAPU).

Financial data can be evaluated as listed on the JHNEBP Nonresearch Evidence Appraisal Tool (Appendix F). When reviewing reports including economic analyses, examine the aim, method, measures, results, and discussion for clarity. Carande-Kulis et al. (2000) recommend that standard inclusion criteria for economic studies have an analytic method and provide sufficient detail regarding the method and results. It is necessary to assess the methodological quality of studies addressing questions about cost-savings and cost-effectiveness (Gomersall et al., 2015). The Community Guide "Economic Evaluation Abstraction Form" (2010), which can be used to assess the quality of economic evaluations, suggests considering the following questions:

- Was the study population well described?
- Was the question being analyzed well defined?
- Did the study define the time frame?
- Were data sources for all costs reported?
- Were data sources and costs appropriate with respect to the program and population being tested?
- Was the primary outcome measure clearly specified?
- Did outcomes include the effects or unintended outcomes of the program?
- Was the analytic model reported in an explicit manner?
- Were sensitivity analyses performed?

When evaluating an article with a cost analysis, it is important to recognize that not all articles that include an economic analysis are strictly financial evaluations. Some may use rigorous research designs and should be appraised using the Research Evidence Appraisal Tool (see Appendix E). For example, a report by Yang, Hung, and Chen (2015) evaluates the impact of different nursing staffing models on patient safety, quality of care, and nursing costs. Three mixed models of nursing staffing, where the portion of nurses compared with nurse aides was 76% (n = 213), 100% (n = 209), and 92% (n = 245), were applied during three different periods between 2006–2010. Results indicated that units with a 76%

proportion of RNs made fewer medication errors and had a lower rate of ventilation weaning, and units with a 92% RN proportion had a lower rate of bloodstream infections. The 76% and 92% RNs groups showed increased urinary tract infection and nursing costs (Yang et al., 2015). After a review of this study, the EBP team would discover that this was actually a descriptive, retrospective cohort design study, which is why use of research appraisal criteria to judge the strength and quality of evidence would be more appropriate.

Program Evaluation (Level V Evidence)

Program evaluation is systematic assessment of all components of a program through the application of evaluation approaches, techniques, and knowledge to improve the planning, implementation, and effectiveness of programs (Chen, 2006). To understand program evaluation, we must first define "program." A *program* has been described as the mechanism and structure used to deliver an intervention or a set of synergistically related interventions (Issel, 2016). Programs can take a variety of forms but have in common the need for thorough planning to identify appropriate interventions and the development of organizational structure in order to effectively implement the program interventions. Monitoring and evaluation should follow so that findings can be used for continued assessment and refinement of the program and its interventions but also to measure the position, validity, and outcomes of the program (Issel, 2016; Whitehead, 2003).

Although program evaluations are commonly conducted within a framework of scientific inquiry and designed as research studies, most internal program evaluations are less rigorous (Level V). Frequently, they comprise pre- or post-implementation data at the organizational level accompanied by qualitative reports of personal satisfaction with the program. For example, in a program evaluation of a patient navigation program, program value and effectiveness were assessed in terms of timeliness of access to cancer care, resolution of barriers, and satisfaction in 55 patients over a six-month period (Koh et al., 2010). While these measures may be helpful in assessing this particular program, they are not standard, accepted measures that serve as benchmarks; thus, close consideration of the methods and findings is crucial for the EBP team when considering this type of evidence (AHRQ, 2018).

Expert Opinion (Level V Evidence)

Expert opinions are another potential source of valuable information. Consisting of views or judgments by subject matter experts and based on their combined knowledge and experience in a particular topic area, these can include case reports, commentary articles, podcasts, written or oral correspondence, and letters to the editor or "op-ed" pieces. Assessing the quality of this evidence requires the EBP team do their due diligence in vetting the author's expert status. Characteristics to consider include education and training, existing body of work, professional and academic affiliations, and their previous publications and communications in the area of interest. For instance, is the author recognized by state, regional, national, or international groups for their expertise? To what degree have their publications been cited by others? Do they have a history of being invited to give lectures or speak at conferences about the issue? One exemplar is an article by Davidson and Rahman (2019), who share their expert opinion on the evolving role of the Clinical Nurse Specialist (CNS) in critical care. This article could be rated as high quality, because they are both experienced CNSs, are doctoral-prepared, belong to several well-established professional organizations, and are leaders in their respective specialties.

Case Report (Level V Evidence)

Case reports are among the oldest forms of medical scholarship and, although appreciation for them has waxed and waned over time (Nissen & Wynn, 2014), they are recently seeing a revival (Bradley, 2018). Providing clinical description of a particular patient, visit, or encounter, case reports can help support development of clinicians' judgment, critical thinking, and decision-making (Oermann & Hays, 2016). They frequently involve unique, interesting, or rare presentations and illustrate successful or unsuccessful care delivery (Porcino, 2016). Multiple case reports can be presented as a case series, comparing and contrasting various aspects of the clinical issue of interest (Porcino, 2016). Case reports and case series are limited in their generalizability, lack controls, and entail selection bias (Sayre et al., 2017), and, being based on experiential and nonresearch evidence, are categorized as Level V.

Case studies, in comparison, are more robust, intensive investigations of a case. They make use of quantitative or qualitative data, can employ statistical analyses, investigate the case of interest over time, or evaluate trends. Thus, case studies are considered quantitative, qualitative, or mixed-methods research (Sandelowski, 2011) and should be evaluated as such. (See Chapter 6 for more information about the different types of research.)

Community Standard (Level V Evidence)

For some EBP topics, it is important to gather information on community practice standards. To do so, the team identifies clinicians, agencies, or organizations to contact for relevant insights, determines their questions, and prepares to collect the data in a systematic manner. There are myriad ways to access communities: email, social media, national or regional conferences, online databases, or professional organization listserv forums. For instance, the Society of Pediatric Nurses has a web-based discussion forum for members to query other pediatric nurses on various practice issues and current standards (http://www.pedsnurses.org/p/cm/ld/fid=148).

In an example of investigating community standards, Johns Hopkins University School of Nursing students were assisting with an EBP project asking: "Does charge nurse availability during the shift affect staff nurse satisfaction with workflow?" An EBP team member contacted local hospitals to determine whether charge nurses had patient assignments. Students developed a data sheet with questions about the healthcare facility, the unit, the staffing pattern, and staff comments about satisfaction. The students reported the number of units contacted and responses, information source, and number of sources using the Nonresearch Evidence Appraisal Tool (Appendix F). Additionally, this approach provided an opportunity to network with other clinicians about a clinical issue.

Clinician Experience (Level V Evidence)

Clinician experience—gained through first-person involvement with and observation of clinical practice—is another possible EBP information source. In the increasingly complex, dynamic healthcare environment, interprofessional teams must work collaboratively to provide safe, high-quality, and cost-effective care. This collaboration allows many opportunities for collegial discussion and sharing of past experiences. Newer clinicians tend to rely more heavily on structured guidelines, protocols, and decision-aids while increasing their practical skillset. With time and exposure to various practice situations, experiences build clinical expertise, allowing for intuitive and holistic understanding of patients and their care needs. When seeking clinician experience to inform an EBP project, the team should evaluate the information source's experiential credibility, the clarity of opinion expressed, and the degree to which evidence from various experienced clinicians is consistent.

Patient/Consumer Experience (Level V Evidence)

Patients are consumers of healthcare, and the term *consumer* also refers to a larger group of individuals using health services in a variety of settings. A patient-centered healthcare model recognizes an individual's unique health needs and desired outcomes as the driving force of all healthcare decisions and quality measurements (NEJM Catalyst, 2017). Patient-centered healthcare expects that patients and families play an active, collaborative, and shared role in decisions, both at an individual level and a system level. Professional organizations and healthcare institutions are increasingly incorporating patient and family expertise into guidelines and program development. Guidelines that do not recognize the importance of the patient's lived experience are set up to fail when the guidelines do not meet the needs of patients and families. Unique characteristics related to personal and cultural values shape an individual's experience of health and their goals for health (DelVecchio Good & Hannah, 2015).

The expert healthcare provider incorporates patient preferences into clinical decision-making by asking the following questions:

- Are the research findings and nonresearch evidence relevant to this particular patient's care?
- Have all care and treatment options based on the best available evidence been presented to the patient?

- Has the patient been given as much time as necessary to allow for clarification and consideration of options?
- Have the patient's expressed preferences and concerns been considered when planning care?

The answer to these questions requires ethical practice and respect for a patient's autonomy. Healthcare providers should also carefully assess the patient/family's level of understanding and provide additional information or resources if needed. Combining sensitivity to and understanding of individual patient needs and thoughtful application of best evidence leads to optimal patient-centered outcomes. The mission of the Patient-Centered Outcomes Research Institute (PCORI), established by the Affordable Care Act 2010, is to "help people make informed healthcare decisions, and improve healthcare delivery and outcomes, by producing and promoting high-integrity, evidence-based information that comes from research guided by patients, caregivers, and the broader healthcare community" (PCORI, n.d., para. 2). To achieve this goal, PCORI engages stakeholders (including patients, clinicians, researchers, payers, industry, purchasers, hospitals and healthcare systems, policymakers, and educators) into the components of comparative-effectiveness research through stakeholder input, consultation, collaboration, and shared leadership (PCORI, n.d.).

Engaging consumers of healthcare in EBP goes beyond individual patient encounters. Consumer organizations can play a significant role in supporting implementation and utilization of EBP. Consumer-led activities can take the form of facilitating research to expedite equitable adoption of new and existing best practices, promoting policies for the development and use of advocacy tool kits, and influencing provider adoption of EBP (DelVecchio Good & Hannah, 2015). Many consumer organizations focus on patient safety initiatives, such as Campaign Zero and preventable hospital harms, or the Josie King Foundation and medical errors. In examining the information provided by consumers, the EBP team should consider the credibility of the individual or group. What segment and volume of the consumer group do they represent? Do their comments and opinions provide any insight into your EBP question?

Best Practices Companies

A relatively recent addition to sources of evidence and best practices are companies that provide consultative business development services. One example, founded in 1979, is The Advisory Board Company; the current mission is to improve healthcare by providing evidence and strategies for implementing best practices (Advisory Board, 2020). The Advisory Board Company has many specific subgroups based on clinical specialty (e.g., cardiovascular, oncology, imaging) and professions (physician executive and nursing executive, among others). Membership allows access to a wide variety of resources, including best practices research, strategic and leadership consultation, and organizational benchmarking using proprietary databases (Advisory Board, 2020). Benefits of utilizing this type of data in development of EBP are the power of collective, international experiences and the ability to source data from one's own institution, but EBP teams should also consider the cost of membership as well as the inherent focus on organizational efficiency, which may lead to some degree of bias.

Recommendations for Healthcare Leaders

Time and resource constraints compel leaders to find creative ways to support integration of new knowledge into clinical practice. The amount of time the average staff member must devote to gathering and appraising evidence is limited. Therefore, finding the most efficient way to gain new knowledge should be a goal of EBP initiatives. Healthcare leaders should not only support staff education initiatives that teach how to read and interpret nonresearch evidence but also become familiar themselves with desired attributes of such information so that they can serve as credible mentors in the change process.

Another challenge for clinicians is to combine the contributions of the two evidence types (research and nonresearch) in making patient care decisions. According to Melnyk and Fineout-Overholt (2006), no "magic bullet" or standard formula exists with which to determine how much weight should be applied to each of these factors when making patient care decisions. It is not sufficient to apply a standard rating system that grades the strength and quality of evidence without determining whether recommendations made by the best evidence are compatible with the patient's values and preferences and the clinician's expertise. Healthcare leaders can best support EBP by providing clinicians with the knowledge and skills necessary to appraise quantitative and qualitative research evidence within the context of nonresearch evidence. Only through continuous learning can clinicians and care teams gain the confidence needed to incorporate the broad range of evidence into the more targeted care of individual patients.

Summary

This chapter describes nonresearch evidence and strategies for evaluating this evidence and recommends approaches for building clinicians' capacity to appraise nonresearch evidence to inform their practice. Nonresearch evidence includes summaries of evidence (clinical practice guidelines, consensus or position statements, literature reviews); organizational experience (quality improvement and financial data); expert opinion (individual commentary or opinion, case reports); community standards; clinician experience; and consumer experience. This evidence includes important information for practice decision. For example, consumer preference is an essential element of the EBP process with increased focus on patient-centered care. In summary, although nonresearch evidence does not have the rigor of research evidence, it does provide important information for informed practice decisions.

References

Abrahamson, K. A., Fox, R. L., & Doebbeling, B. N. (2012). Facilitators and barriers to clinical practice guideline use among nurses. *American Journal of Nursing, 12*(7), 26–35. https://doi.org/10.1097/01.NAJ.0000415957.46932.bf

Advisory Board. (2020). *About us*. https://www.advisory.com/en/about-us

Agency for Healthcare Research and Quality. (2018). *Patient self-management support programs: An evaluation*. https://www.ahrq.gov/research/findings/final-reports/ptmgmt/evaluation.html

The AGREE Research Trust. (2013). *The AGREE II instrument*. http://www.agreetrust.org/wp-content/uploads/2013/10/AGREE-II-Users-Manual-and-23-item-Instrument_2009_UPDATE_2013.pdf

Alonso-Coello, P., Irfan, A., Sola, I., Delgado-Noguera, M., Rigau, D., Tort, S., Bonfil, X., Burgers, J., Shunemann H. (2010). The quality of clinical practice guidelines over the past two decades: A systematic review of guideline appraisal studies. *BMJ Quality & Safety, 19*(6), e58. doi:10.1136/qshc.2010.042077

Altman, D. G., & Simera, I. (2016). A history of the evolution of guidelines for reporting medical research: The long road to the EQUATOR Network. *Journal of the Royal Society of Medicine, 109*(2), 67–77. https://doi.org/10.1177/0141076815625599

Baker, K. M., Clark, P. R., Henderson, D., Wolf, L. A., Carman, M. J., Manton, A., & Zavotsky, K. E. (2014). Identifying the differences between quality improvement, evidence-based practice, and original research. *Journal of Emergency Nursing, 40*(2), 195–197. https://doi.org/10.1016/j.jen.2013.12.016

Bradley, P. J. (2018). Guidelines to authors publishing a case report: The need for quality improvement. *ACR Case Reports, 2*(4). https://doi.org/10.21037/acr.2018.04.02

Brouwers, M. C., Kho, M. E., Browman, G. P., Burgers, J. S., Cluzeau, F., Feder, G., Fervers, B., Graham, I. D., Hanna, S. E., & Makarski, J. (2010). Development of the AGREE II, part 1: Performance, usefulness and areas for improvement. *Canadian Medical Association Journal, 182*(10), 1045–1062. https://doi.org/10.1503/cmaj.091714

Carande-Kulis, V. G., Maciosek, M. V., Briss, P. A., Teutsch, S. M., Zaza, S., Truman, B. I., Messonnier, M. L., Pappaioanou, M., Harris, J. R., & Fielding, J. (2000). Methods for systematic reviews of economic evaluations for the guide to community preventive service. *American Journal of Preventive Medicine, 18*(1S), 75–91. https://doi.org/10.1016/s0749-3797(99)00120-8

Carper, B. A. (1978). Fundamental patterns of knowing in nursing. *ANS Advances in Nursing Science, 1*(1), 13–24. https://doi.org/10.1097/00012272-197810000-00004

Carter, E. J., Mastro, K., Vose, C., Rivera, R., & Larson, E. L. (2017). Clarifying the conundrum: Evidence-based practice, quality improvement, or research? The clinical scholarship continuum. *Journal of Nursing Administration, 47*(5), 266–270. https://doi.org/10.1097/NNA.0000000000000477

Centers for Disease Control and Prevention. (2007). *Economic evaluation of public health preparedness and response efforts.* http://www.cdc.gov/owcd/EET/SeriesIntroduction/TOC.html

Chen, H. T. (2006). A theory-driven evaluation perspective on mixed methods research. *Res Sch, 13*(1), 75–83.

Cohen, R. I., Kennedy, H., Amitrano, B., Dillon, M., Guigui, S., & Kanner, A. (2015). A quality improvement project to decrease emergency department and medical intensive care unit transfer times. *Journal of Critical Care, 30*(6), 1331–1337. https://doi.org/10.1016/j.jcrc.2015.07.017

Community Guide economic evaluation abstraction form, Version 4.0. (2010). https://www.thecommunityguide.org/sites/default/files/assets/EconAbstraction_v5.pdf

Conn, V. S. (2004). Meta-analysis research. *Journal of Vascular Nursing, 22*(2), 51–52. https://doi.org/10.1016/j.jvn.2004.03.002

Connelly, L. (2018). Overview of quality improvement. *MEDSURG Nursing, 27*(2), 125–126.

Dahm, P., Yeung, L. L., Galluci, M., Simone, G., & Schunemann, H. J. (2009). How to use a clinical practice guideline. *The Journal of Urology, 181*(2), 472–479. https://doi.org/10.1016/j.juro.2008.10.041

Davidson, P. M., & Rahman, A. R. (2019). Time for a renaissance of the clinical nurse specialist role in critical care? *AACN Advanced Critical Care*, *30*(1), 61–64. https://doi.org/10.4037/aacnacc2019779

DelVecchio Good, M.-J., & Hannah, S. D. (2015). "Shattering culture": Perspectives on cultural competence and evidence-based practice in mental health services. *Transcultural Psychiatry*, *52*(2), 198–221. https://doi.org/10.1177/1363461514557348

Diekemper, R. L., Patel, S., Mette, S. A., Ornelas, J., Ouellette, D. R., Casey, K. R. (2018). Making the GRADE: CHEST updates its methodology. *Chest*, *153*(3), 756–759. https://doi.org/10.1016/j.chest.2016.04.018

Emergency Care Research Institute (ECRI). 2020. https://guidelines.ecri.org/about-trust-scorecard/

EQUATOR Network. (n.d.). *Reporting guidelines for main study types*. EQUATOR Network: Enhancing the QUAlity and Transparency of Health Research. https://www.equator-network.org

Fervers, B., Burgers, J. S., Haugh, M. C., Brouwers, M., Browman, G., Cluzeau, F., & Philip, T. (2005). Predictors of high quality clinical practice guidelines: Examples in oncology. *International Journal for Quality in Health Care*, *17*(2), 123–132. https://doi.org/10.1093/intqhc/mzi011

Gomersall, J. S., Jadotte, Y. T., Xue, Y., Lockwood S., Riddle D., & Preda, A. (2015). Conducting systematic reviews of economic evaluations. *International Journal of Evidence Based Healthcare*, *13*(3), 170–178. https://doi.org/10.1097/XEB.0000000000000063

Grant, M. J., & Booth, A. (2009). A typology of reviews: An analysis of 14 review types and associated methodologies. *Health Information and Libraries Journal*, *26*(2), 91–108. https://doi.org/10.1111/j.1471-1842.2009.00848.x

Gray, A. M., & Wilkinson, T. (2106). Economic evaluation of healthcare interventions: Old and new directions. *Oxford Review of Economic Policy*, *32*(1), 102–121.

Institute of Medicine. (2011). *Clinical practice guidelines we can trust*. The National Academies Press. Retrieved from http://www.nationalacademies.org/hmd/Reports/2011/Clinical-Practice-Guidelines-We-Can-Trust/Standards.aspx

Issel, L. M. (2016). Health program planning and evaluation: What nurse scholars need to know. In J. R. Bloch, M. R. Courtney, & M. L. Clark (Eds.), *Practice-based clinical inquiry in nursing for DNP and PhD research: Looking beyond traditional methods* (1st ed.), 3–16. Springer Publishing Company.

Joshi, G. P, Benzon, H. T, Gan, T. J., & Vetter, T. R. (2019). Consistent definitions of clinical practice guidelines, consensus statements, position statements, and practice alerts. *Anesthesia & Analgesia*, *129*(6), 1767–1769. https://doi.org/10.1213/ANE.0000000000004236

Koh, C., Nelson, J. M., & Cook, P. F. (2010). Evaluation of a patient navigation program. *Clinical Journal of Oncology Nursing*, *15*(1), 41–48. https://doi.org/10.1188/11.CJON.41-48

Kuehn, B. M. (2011). IOM sets out "gold standard" practices for creating guidelines, systematic reviews. *JAMA*, *305*(18), 1846–1848.

Lopez-Olivo, M. A., Kallen, M. A., Ortiz, Z., Skidmore, B., & Suarez-Almazor, M. E. (2008). Quality appraisal of clinical practice guidelines and consensus statements on the use of biologic agents in rheumatoid arthritis: A systematic review. *Arthritis & Rheumatism*, *59*(11), 1625–1638. https://doi.org/10.1002/art.24207

Melnyk, B. M., & Fineout-Overholt, E. (2006). Consumer preferences and values as an integral key to evidence-based practice. *Nursing Administration Quarterly, 30*(2), 123–127. https://doi.org/10.1097/00006216-200604000-00009

Mims, J. W. (2015). Targeting quality improvement in clinical practice guidelines. *Otolaryngology— Head and Neck Surgery, 153*(6), 907–908. https://doi.org/10.1177/0194599815611861

NEJM Catalyst. (2017, January 1). What is patient-centered care? *NEJM Catalyst.* https://catalyst.nejm.org/doi/abs/10.1056/CAT.17.0559

Neumann, I., Santesso, N., Akl, E. A., Rind, D. M., Vandvik, P. O., Alonso-Coello, P., Agoritsas, T., Mustafa, R. A., Alexander, P. E., Schünemann, H., & Guyatt, G. H. (2016). A guide for health professionals to interpret and use recommendations in guidelines developed with the GRADE approach. *Journal of Clinical Epidemiology, 72*, 45–55. https://doi.org/10.1016/j.jclinepi.2015.11.017

Newhouse, R. P., Pettit, J. C., Poe, S., & Rocco, L. (2006). The slippery slope: Differentiating between quality improvement and research. *Journal of Nursing Administration, 36*(4), 211–219. https://doi.org/10.1097/00005110-200604000-00011

Nissen, S. E. (2017). Conflicts of interest and professional medical associations: Progress and remaining challenges. *JAMA, 317*(17), 1737–1738. https://doi.org/10.1001/jama.2017.2516

Nissen, T., & Wynn, R. (2014). The clinical case report: a review of its merits and limitations. *BMC research notes, 7*, 264. https://doi.org/10.1186/1756-0500-7-264

Oermann, M. H., & Hays, J. C. (2016). *Writing for publication in nursing* (3rd ed.). Springer.

Ogrinc, G., Davies, L., Baltalden, P., Davidoff, F., Goodman, D., & Stevens, D. (2015). *SQUIRE 2.0.* http://www.squire-statement.org

Patient-Centered Outcomes Research Institute. (n.d.). *Our vision & mission.* https://www.pcori.org/about-us/our-vision-mission

Peters, M. D. J., Godfrey, C. M., Khalil, H., McInerny, P., Parker, D., & Soares, C. B. (2015). Guidance for conducting systematic scoping reviews. *International Journal of Evidence-Based Healthcare, 13*(3), 141–146. https://doi.org/10.1097/xeb.0000000000000050

Porcino, A. (2016). Not birds of a feather: Case reports, case studies, and single-subject research. *International Journal of Therapeutic Massage & Bodywork, 9*(3), 1–2. https://doi.org/10.3822/ijtmb.v9i3.334

Portela, M. C., Pronovost, P. J., Woodcock, T., Carter, P., & Dixon-Woods, M. (2015). How to study improvement interventions: A brief overview of possible study types. *BMJ Quality and Safety, 24*(5), 325–336. https://doi.org/10.1136/bmjqs-2014-003620

Ransohoff, D. F., Pignone, M., & Sox, H. C. (2013). How to decide whether a clinical practice guideline is trustworthy. *Journal of the American Medical Association, 309*(2), 139–140. https://doi.org/10.1001/jama.2012.156703

Sandelowski, M. (2011), "Casing" the research case study. *Res. Nurs. Health, 34:* 153-159. https://doi.org/10.1002/nur.20421

Sayre, J. W., Toklu, H. Z., Ye, F., Mazza, J., & Yale, S. (2017). Case reports, case series—From clinical practice to evidence-based medicine in graduate medical education. *Cureus, 8*(8), e1546. https://doi.org/10.7759/cureus.1546

Senn, S. J. (2009). Overstating the evidence—Double counting in meta-analysis and related problems. *BMC Medical Research Methodology, 9*, 10. https://doi.org/10.1186/1471-2288-9-10

Shekelle, P. G. (2018). Clinical practice guidelines: What's next? *JAMA, 320*(8), 757–758. https://doi.org/10.1001/jama.2018.9660

Sniderman, A. D., & Furberg, C. D. (2009). Why guideline-making requires reform. *Journal of the American Medical Association, 301*(4), 429–431. https://doi.org/10.1001/jama.2009.15

Snyder, H. (2019). Literature review as a research methodology: An overview and guidelines. *Journal of Business Research, 104*, 333–339. https://doi.org/10.1016/j.jbusres.2019.07.039

Spetz, J., Brown, D. S., Aydin, C., & Donaldson, N. (2013). The value of reducing hospital-acquired pressure ulcer prevalence: An illustrative analysis. *Journal of Nursing Administration, 43*(4), 235–241. https://doi.org/10.1097/NNA.0b013e3182895a3c

Stetler, C. B., Morsi, D., Rucki, S., Broughton, S., Corrigan, B., Fitzgerald, J., Giuliano, K., Havener, P., & Sheridan, E. A. (1998). Utilization-focused integrative reviews in a nursing service. *Applied Nursing Research, 11*(4), 195–206. https://doi.org/10.1016/s0897-1897(98)80329-7

Sullivan, T. (2018, May 5). Physicians and industry: Fix the relationships but keep them going. *Policy & Medicine.* https://www.policymed.com/2011/02/physicians-and-industry-fix-the-relationships-but-keep-them-going.html

Toronto, C. E., Quinn, B. L., & Remington, R. (2018). Characteristics of reviews published in nursing literature. *Advances in Nursing Science, 41*(1), 30–40. https://doi.org/10.1097/ANS.0000000000000180

Tunkel, D. E., & Jones, S. L. (2015). Who wrote this clinical practice guideline? *Otolaryngology-Head and Neck Surgery, 153*(6), 909–913. https://doi.org/10.1177/0194599815606716

Welch, V. A., Akl, E. A., Guyatt, G., Pottie, K., Eslava-Schmalbach, J., Ansari, M. T., de Beer, H., Briel, M., Dans, T., Dans, I., Hultcrantz, M., Jull, J., Katikireddi, S. V., Meerpohl, J., Morton, R., Mosdol, A., Petkovic, J., Schünemann, H. J., Sharaf, R. N., ... Tugwell, P. (2017). GRADE equity guidelines 1: Considering health equity in GRADE guideline development: introduction and rationale. *Journal of Clinical Epidemiology, 90*, 59–67. https://doi.org/10.1016/j.jclinepi.2017.01.014

Whitehead, D. (2003). Evaluating health promotion: A model for nursing practice. *Journal of Advanced Nursing, 41*(5), 490–498. https://doi.org/10.1046/j.1365-2648.2003.02556.x

Whittemore, R. (2005). Combining evidence in nursing research: Methods and implications. *Nursing Research, 54*(1), 56–62. https://doi.org/10.1097/00006199-200501000-00008

Whittemore, R., & Knafl, K. (2005). The integrative review: Updated methodology. *Journal of Advanced Nursing, 52*(5), 546–553. https://doi.org/10.1111/j.1365-2648.2005.03621.x

Yang, P. H., Hung, C. H., & Chen, Y. C. (2015). The impact of three nursing staffing models on nursing outcomes. *Journal of Advanced Nursing, 71*(8), 1847–1856. https://doi.org/10.1111/jan.12643

Yoder-Wise, P. S. (2014). *Leading and managing in nursing* (6th ed.). Mosby.

Translation

The final phase of the PET process is translation, the value-added step in evidence-based practice. Translation leads to a change in practice, processes, or systems and in the resulting outcomes. Through translation, the EBP team assesses the best evidence recommendations identified in the Evidence phase for transferability to a desired practice setting; followed by implementation, evaluation, and communication of practice changes. This chapter covers the Translation phase of the PET process and will:

- Examine evidence criteria that determine recommendation(s) for implementation
- Review organization-specific considerations essential to translation of best evidence
- Specify the components of an action plan
- Identify steps in implementing and evaluating a practice change

Implementation of best evidence is the primary reason to conduct an evidence review. Critically appraising, rating, and grading existing evidence and making practice recommendations requires one set of skills; translation requires another.

The EBP process requires both critical thinking and clinical reasoning. Critical thinking, a key skill or process integral for clinical reasoning, is knowledge-based and is not dependent on the specific patient, situation, or environment (Victor-Chmil, 2013). While critical thinking is an essential component of the Evidence phase of the PET process, clinical reasoning is the essential component of the Translation phase. Clinical reasoning, a set of cognitive processes, requires clinicians to identify the relevance of the evidence and knowledge to a particular patient, situation, or setting. Thus, the EBP team engages in clinical reasoning to evaluate the relevance of the best evidence recommendations to their practice setting (Kuiper & Pesut, 2004; Victor-Chmil, 2013).

Before we describe the translation process, it is important to clarify some terminology used in translation. Study or project teams often use the terms *translation* and *implementation* interchangeably, which is appropriate; however, we describe the significant difference between translation and implementation science (see Box 8.1).

Translation Models

The use of a translation model or framework in this phase of the PET process is imperative in ensuring a systematic and intentional approach to the change. First and foremost, the team selects a model or framework to ensure a fully realized translation. There are multiple frameworks or models to choose from; Tabak et al. (2012) reviewed sixty-one current translation models. Many focus on implementing evidence into practice, enhanced by a body of literature that describes implementation strategies (Waltz et al., 2015). Secondly, translation requires organizational support, human and material resources, and a commitment of individuals and interprofessional teams. Context, communication, leadership, mentoring, and evidence affect the implementation and dissemination of best evidence into practice. Finally, planning and active coordination by the team are critical to successful translation, as is adherence to principles of change that guide this process and careful attention to the characteristics of the organization involved (Newhouse et al., 2007; White et al., 2020).

> **Box 8.1 Implementation Science**
>
> *Implementation science* is "the scientific study of methods to promote the systematic uptake of research findings and other evidence-based practices into routine practice, and, hence, to improve the quality and effectiveness of health services and care" (Eccles & Mittman, 2006, p. 1). Implementation science tries to understand how, when, where, and why change processes work. By rigorously studying methods of systems improvements, they attempt to answer the question: What are the best methods to facilitate the uptake of evidence into practice?
>
> Over the last 20 years, there has been concern that local success in translating evidence into practice is often challenging to replicate, spread, and sustain. Factors that facilitate the change in practice may work in one setting but not in another. These local successes, performed in a single setting of convenience, are not generalizable because the translation does not consider other critical organizational contributing or confounding factors. In addition, simplistic impact measures are often used, and spread and sustainability are rarely part of the translation strategy. Implementation science focuses on researching the efficacy and effectiveness of different translation strategies and the rigorous testing of improvement strategies. Well-designed and effective implementation strategies affect the sustainability of those efforts (White et al., 2020).

We describe The Model for Improvement: PDSA (Langley et al., 2009) to translate evidence into practice because it is one of the most used and successful translation approaches in healthcare. In addition to the PDSA cycle, other models (see Table 8.1) may be more appropriate given the complexity and scale of change being implemented.

Table 8.1   Models and Frameworks for Translation and Implementation of Evidence

Model or Framework	Description	Best Used For
AHRQ: Knowledge Transfer	Accelerates the transfer of research findings to organizations that can benefit from it. Includes three phases: 1) knowledge creation and distillation, 2) diffusion and dissemination, and 3) end user adoption (Nieva et al., 2005).	Developing tools and strategies to implement research findings, specifically for AHRQ grantees and healthcare providers engaged in direct patient care to improve care quality (Nieva et al., 2005).
Knowledge-to-Action	Integrates creation and application of knowledge. Knowledge creation includes knowledge inquiry, synthesis, and tools/products; knowledge becomes more refined as it moves through these three steps. Action includes identifying and appraising the problem and the known research; identifying barriers and successes; planning and executing; and finally monitoring, evaluating, and adjusting (Graham, 2006).	Facilitating the use of research knowledge by several stakeholders, such as practitioners, policymakers, patients, and the public (Graham et al., 2006).
PARIHS	Examines the interactions between evidence, context, and facilitation to translate evidence into practice by placing equal importance on the setting and how the evidence is introduced into the setting as well as the quality of the evidence itself (Bergström et al., 2020).	Organizing framework to specify determinants that act as barriers and enablers influencing implementation outcomes (Bergström et al., 2020).

QUERI Implementation Roadmap to Implement Evidence-Based Practices	Drives the adoption of high-value research innovations by empowering frontline providers, researchers, administrators, and health system leaders by focusing on the development of practical products (e.g., implementation playbook) and a data-driven evaluation plan (Stetler et al., 2008).	Based on quality improvement science, is distinctively suited for use in real-world settings to support further scale-up and spread of an effective practice (Stetler et al., 2008).
RE-AIM	Designed to enhance the quality, speed, and public health impact of efforts to translate research into practice in five steps: ■ **R**each your intended target population ■ **E**fficacy (or effectiveness) ■ **A**doption by target staff, settings, systems, or communities ■ **I**mplementation consistency, costs, and adaptations made during delivery ■ **M**aintenance of intervention effects in individuals and settings over time (Glasgow et al., 1999)	Determine public health impact, translate research into practice, help plan programs and improve their chances of working in "real-world" settings, and understand the relative strengths and weaknesses of different approaches to health promotion and chronic disease self-management—such as in-person counseling, group education classes, telephone counseling, and internet resources (Glasgow et al., 1999).

Notes: QUERI – Quality Enhancement Research Initiative; PARIHS – Promoting Action on Research Implementation in Health Services

The Model for Improvement: PDSA

The Plan-Do-Study-Act (PDSA) cycle is a four-stage quality improvement (QI) model. PDSA approaches are simple, rapid cycle quality improvement processes that provide a structured, data-driven learning approach that allows teams to assess whether a change leads to improvement in a particular setting and to make appropriate, timely adjustments. PDSA uses a "test of change" approach to quickly troubleshoot issues as well as increase the scale and complexity of the translation to achieve the desired improvement. To properly implement and evaluate the cycles, the EBP team must form a translation team. This translation team may be different from the original team that evaluated the evidence due to the need to include team members who can identify and address any problems in the specific local context where the evidence is implemented.

The translation team sets measurable goals and integrates measurement into daily workflows. Goal setting includes drafting aims using the SMART goal format (Table 8.2) and establishing measures to assess change.

Table 8.2   Definition of a SMART Goal

Specific	Goals should be straightforward and state what you want to happen. Be specific and define what you are going to do. Use action words such as *direct, organize, coordinate, lead, develop, plan,* etc.
Measurable	If you can't measure it, you can't manage it. Choose goals with measurable progress, and establish concrete criteria for measuring the success of your goal.
Achievable	Goals must be within your capacity to reach. If goals are set too far out of your reach, you cannot commit to accomplishing them. A goal should stretch you slightly so you feel you can do it, and it will need a real commitment from you. Success in reaching attainable goals keeps you motivated.
Relevant	Goals should be relevant. Make sure each goal is consistent with your other goals and aligned with the goals of the company, your manager, or your department.
Time-bound	Set a time frame for the goal: for next week, in three months, end of the quarter. Putting an end point on your goal gives you a clear target to work toward. Without a time limit, there's no urgency to start taking action now.

Source: Johns Hopkins Performance Evaluation Resource

For successful data collection of the identified measures, a simple data collection form may be beneficial, as well as assigning data collection into daily tasks (preferably of one or two point people). The PDSA process requires the team to answer three fundamental questions, in any order (Figure 8.1): What are we trying to accomplish? How will we know that a change is an improvement? What change can we make that will result in an improvement?

To answer these questions, the team engages in four stages that compose the PDSA model (Table 8.3).

Table 8.3 Plan-Do-Study-Act Model Stages and Definitions

Stages	Activity	Definition
I	Plan	Develop a plan to test the change that answers the questions: What data will the team collect? Who? What? When? Where?
II	Do	Carry out the plan and document unexpected problems and observations.
III	Study	Analyze and study the results, summarize, and reflect on learning(s).
IV	Act	Define the change based on what was learned from the test, and determine what modifications should be made.

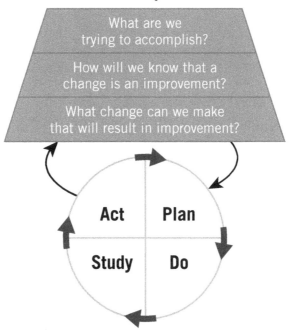

Figure 8.1 Model for Improvement.

Components of the Translation Phase

Component 1: Identify Practice Setting–Specific Recommendations

The translation phase begins when the interprofessional practice team selects a course of action to implement a change or pilot (Appendix I) and agrees on the organization-specific recommendations. Critical to the translation are the relationships of this interprofessional team that capitalize on the knowledge and skills that each member brings, including an understanding of the specific practice setting. The team takes responsibility for translation of the best evidence to the local context. Translation requires that the team assess the fit, feasibility, and acceptability of the recommendations within the organization's context (White et al., 2020).

Component 2: Determine Fit, Feasibility, and Acceptability of Recommendations to the Organization

Practice recommendations made in the evidence phase, even if based on compelling evidence, might not be suitable to implement in all settings. The EBP team is responsible for evaluating best evidence recommendations for implementation within the practice setting (see Appendix I). Stetler (2001, 2010) recommends using specific criteria such as fit, feasibility, and desirability.

Assessment of the *fit* to the current practice environment involves consideration of the extent to which the change is suited to the end user's workflow and if the change sufficiently improves a specific practice problem. The EBP team accomplishes this by evaluating the current environment, the extent to which the change aligns with organizational priorities, and the infrastructure in place, such as resources (equipment or products) and the presence of people who can foster change or facilitate the adoption of the evidence (Greenhalgh et al., 2004).

Determining the *feasibility* of implementing best evidence recommendations within an organizational setting involves assessing the extent to which the team evaluates and believes the change is doable, that barriers are realistic to overcome, and that risk is minimal. The team should assess the practice environment's readiness for change, which includes the availability of human and material resources, support from decision-makers (individuals and groups), and budget implications; and they evaluate and determine whether it is possible to develop strategies to overcome barriers to implementation. Strategies include seeking input and involvement from the frontline staff, stakeholders, and other individuals affected by the change and cocreating communication, education, and implementation plans with those most affected by the change. The final area to assess for feasibility before implementing proposed recommendations is to evaluate the risk of making the change in the specific practice environment. This risk assessment focuses on identifying, analyzing, and discussing safety vulnerabilities that the change may create for the organization. A Heat Chart is a useful quality improvement tool that shows a visual or graphical picture of complex dimensions of problems, or in this case, the risk consideration during the action planning steps for translation. Figure 8.2 provides a color-coded stop light representation of the interrelated role of risk and strength and consistency of evidence when the team is determining whether best evidence should be put into practice. (NOTE: The ebook versions of this book present the heat chart in color with reds, yellows, and greens, while the print book presents the same information using black, gray, and white indicating "stop," "use caution," and "proceed," respectively.) Interventions with higher risks require more strong, consistent, and compelling evidence than those with lower risks. It is also important to note, that although an intervention with little or conflicting evidence may be low risk, it should still be translated judiciously to ensure the team is not wasting time and resources on a change not supported by the literature.

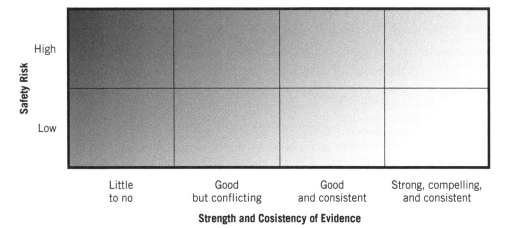

Figure 8.2 Heat chart for interconnected role of safety risk and strength and consistency of best evidence.

The final area to consider is that of acceptability. *Acceptability* refers to the extent to which stakeholders and organizational leadership perceive the EBP change to be agreeable and palatable, and trust that the change is reasonable. Leadership is a critical element in the effective implementation of innovations and change within an organization (Aarons et al., 2015). EBP teams should seek opportunities to inform key stakeholders and leaders within the organization about their progress to obtain their input and feedback throughout the PET process. Key collaborators include leaders in areas such as organizational risk management, quality improvement, and patient safety. Keeping these leaders and leaders of the target change area(s) informed positions the team for organizational support during implementation of recommended changes and increases the likelihood of change adoption and sustainability.

In summary, change initiatives such as translation are prone to failure and waste valuable time and resources on efforts that produce negligible benefits when the assessment of safety risk; quality of the best evidence; availability of resources, including money, time, and staff; and other factors that could negatively impact the translation are not considered during this action planning phase.

Component 3: Create an Action Plan for Translation

Creating an action plan, informed by a translation model or framework, provides manageable steps to implement change and assigns responsibility for carrying the project forward. The translation team develops specific strategies to introduce, promote, support, and evaluate the practice change. It can be helpful to formulate the plan in a template that includes a timeline with progress columns (see Appendix I).

The action plan includes:

- Development of the strategy for translation of the change (e.g., protocol, guideline, system, or process)
- Specification of a detailed timeline, assignment of team members to high-level task categories and subtasks, an evaluation process, and a plan for how results will be reported
- Solicitation of feedback on the action plan from organizational leadership, bedside clinicians, and other stakeholders

The action plan begins with validation of the determination of fit, feasibility, and acceptability for translation to the specific practice setting and the readiness of the unit, department, or organization for change. Organizational infrastructure is the cornerstone of successful translation. Infrastructure provides human and material resources that are fundamental in preparation for change (Greenhalgh et al., 2004; Newhouse & White, 2011). Readiness for translation includes assessing the current state and strategically planning for building the capacity of the organization before implementation begins. Additionally, fully realized translation requires organizational resources and commitment. Paying particular attention to the planning and implementation of organization-specific recommendations can improve the potential for successfully meeting the project's goals. Beyond human and material readiness, teams need to consider organizational/department/unit culture.

Organizational culture refers to group-learned attitudes, beliefs, and assumptions as the unit, department, or organization integrates and adapts to internal and external forces. These attitudes, beliefs, and assumptions become attributes of the group and subsequently become the preferred way to "perceive, think, and feel in relation to problems" (Schein, 2004, p. 17). To change the culture, the team must challenge tradition, reinforce the need for evidence to inform decisions, and change old patterns of behavior, which sometimes requires new skills. Additional detail and tools to assess organizational readiness and culture are available elsewhere (Poe & White, 2010).

Johns Hopkins Nursing uses one strategy extensively to effectively manage and work through the human side of organizational change. Bridges and Bridges (2017) model, *Managing Transitions: Making the Most of Change*, suggests the Four Ps—Purpose, Picture, Plan, Part (see Table 8.4)—to give those affected by the change time and opportunity to internalize the change and a forum to express their questions or concerns. Those who are outspoken about the change are often those who genuinely care about getting things right and can recognize the pitfalls and make great suggestions to improve the planning activities.

Table 8.4   Four Ps Tool to Communicate Change

Purpose Why are we making this change?	Share with others who are not involved in the planning why things are changing and what will happen if things stay the same.
Picture What will it look like?	Share what the desired outcome will look like; invite staff to co-create the picture with you. Paint a picture of how the outcome will look and feel.
Plan What is the plan and path to the end point?	Lay out, step by step, the plan and path to the new state; invite staff to critique, contribute to, and change the path; make an idea list and a worry list.
Part What part will they have in creating the plan and end point?	People own what they create, so let staff know what you need from them, what part they will have, and where they will have choices or input.

Component 4: Secure Support and Resources to Implement Action Plan

To ensure a successful translation (see Appendix A), first appoint a project leader and identify change champions who are supportive of the recommended practice change and who will be able to support the project leader during the translation phase of the project. *Change champions* are individuals within an organization who volunteer or are selected to facilitate the change. The change champion is an active member of the staff who will be involved during the full implementation of the practice change. Once champions are on board, consider whether the translation activities will require any additional skills, knowledge, or individuals who can assist with or will be essential to the success of the work. These additional members, often referred to as *opinion leaders*, are usually well-known individuals to the practice group in the organization whose opinion is held in high esteem and could influence the practice group's perspective for or against the change. The opinion leader is often someone that the group members turn to for advice or views on matters of importance, so it is critical to identify them in the process.

Once this group is organized, its members identify barriers and facilitators to the success of the proposed practice change, surfacing strengths to tap into and use those to overcome the barriers. They consider how the change affects current policies and procedures, the workflow and throughput of the unit or department, and technological supports to the group's usual work, such as the electronic health record (EHR) or another technology that the group depends on.

Securing support from stakeholders and decision-makers is critical to the implementation phase. Availability of funds to cover expenses associated with the translation and the allocation of human, material, and technological resources is dependent on the endorsement of stakeholders, such as organizational leaders or committees and in collaboration with those individuals or groups affected by the recommendations. It may be necessary to bring in content or external experts to consult on the translation. One key milestone in formulating the action plan is an estimation of expenses and resources needed for translation and potential funding sources. Decision-makers may support wide implementation of the change, request a small test of the change to validate effectiveness, request revisions of the plan or recommendations, or reject the implementation plan. Preparing for the presentation or meeting with decision-makers, involving stakeholders (see Appendix C), and creating a comprehensive action plan are the key steps in building organizational support.

The action plan should include identifying critical high-level categories of activities and associated tasks designed to meet the goals of the project to complete the translation. The plan should include SMART goals, a schedule of all necessary activities, and an assignment of who is responsible for each activity and the target time frame for completion. The action plan should also include activities associated with collection and analysis of the pre- and post-measures (see Appendix B) for evaluation of the practice change.

Component 5: Implement the Action Plan

After the EBP team creates the action plan and secures support, implementation begins. The first step is a small test of the change, or *pilot*. The team seeks input from stakeholders and staff affected by the change and communicates the effective date of implementation and the pilot evaluation plan. This communication can take the form of an agenda item at a staff meeting, an in-service, a direct mailing, an email, a bulletin board, or a video, for example. Stakeholders and staff must know who the project leader is, where to access needed information or supplies, and how to communicate to the project leader issues as they arise. The team obtains staff input along the way to identify problems and address them as soon as possible.

Component 6: Evaluate Outcomes

After implementing the change, the EBP team uses the measures identified in the PICO to evaluate the success of the change. Collaborating with the QI experts can be important during the evaluation process for guidance on tools and appropriate intervals to measure the change. Selecting and developing measures includes defining the purpose of measurement, choosing the clinical areas to evaluate, selecting and developing the metrics, and evaluating the results (Pronovost et al., 2001 [adapted from McGlynn, 1998]). The EBP team compares baseline data to post-implementation data to determine whether the change should be implemented on a wider scale. Measures may encompass five types of outcomes (Poe & White, 2010, p. 157); see Table 8.5.

Table 8.5   Five Types of Outcome Measures

Outcomes	Definition
Clinical	Patient- or disease-focused and therefore reflects certain aspects of an illness; they can be physiological (e.g., a lab value), or they can be adverse event-focused (e.g., falls).
Functional	Measures patient responses or their adaptation to health problems; examples include factors such as ability to perform activities of daily living, self-care, or quality of life.

Perceptual	Applies to both the patient and the provider and their self-report of experiences with care or their work environment, for example, their satisfaction; perceptual experiences also include comprehension related to education and the demonstration or application of that knowledge.
Process or Intervention	Measures of the appropriateness of treatment or care, including process measures such as The Joint Commission core measure of blood culture collection prior to antibiotic administration for treatment of pneumonia; other evidence-based process measures include falls prevention, turning to prevent pressure ulcers, and medication reconciliation to prevent medication errors.
Organization, Departmental, Unit-Based	Focuses on administrative factors that provide evidence of effectiveness, or management issues such as staff fatigue related to working greater than three consecutive 12-hour shifts.

Final Steps of the Translation Phase

The Translation Phase needs to include communication to all participants and stakeholders in the translation process. The communication plan should be targeted to the specific audience and can use multiple venues. For example, the transition team provides regular communication about the progress at their unit or department meetings. Additionally, other forms of messaging, such as bulletin boards, posters, or data dashboards, can provide updates. Change champions and opinion leaders are critical assets to getting the updates out to all involved. Finally, targeting the report of the translation results to all stakeholders will require careful planning and discussion by the team. A one-size-fits-all communication strategy will not be successful. The transition team should customize the messages to the specific stakeholders and audiences. Communication and dissemination are discussed in Chapter 9.

Summary

Translation is the value proposition of evidence-based practice. While the PET Phases are linear, the steps in the process may be iterative and generate new questions, recommendations, or actions. The organizational infrastructure needed to support robust translation of best evidence into practice includes budgetary support; human and material resources; and the commitment of individuals, stakeholders, and interprofessional teams. Translation of recommendations requires organizational skills, project management, and leaders with a high level of influence and tenacity.

References

Aarons, G. A., Ehrhart, M. G., Farahnak, L. R., & Hurlburt, M. S. (2015). Leadership and organizational change for implementation (LOCI): A randomized mixed method pilot study of a leadership and organization development intervention for evidence-based practice implementation. *Implementation Science*, *10*(11), 1–12. https://doi.org/10.1186/s13012-014-0192-y

Bergström, A., Ehrenberg, A., Eldh, A. C., Graham, I. D., Gustafsson, K., Harvey, G., Hunter, S., Kitson, A., Rycroft-Malone, J., & Wallin, L. (2020). The use of the PARIHS framework in implementation research and practice—A citation analysis of the literature. *Implementation Science*, *15*(1), 1–51. https://doi.org/10.1186/s13012-020-01003-0

Bridges, W., & Bridges, S. M. (2017). *Managing transitions: Making the most of change* (4th ed.). Da Capo Lifelong Books.

Eccles, M. P., & Mittman, B. S. *Welcome to Implementation Science. Implementation Sci*1,1 (2006). https://doi.org/10.1186/1748-5908-1-1

Eccles, M. P., Lavis, J. N., Hill, S. J., & Squires, J. E. (2012). Knowledge translation of research findings. *Implementation Science*, *7*(50). https://doi.org/10.1186/1748-5908-7-50

Glasgow, R. E., Vogt, T. M., & Boles, S. M. (1999). Evaluating the public health impact of health promotion interventions: The RE-AIM framework. *American Journal of Public Health*, *89*(9), 1322–1327. https://doi.org/10.2105/AJPH.89.9.1322

Graham, I. D., Logan, J., Harrison, M. B., Straus, S. E., Tetroe, J., Caswell, W., & Robinson, N. (2006). Lost in knowledge translation: Time for a map? *Journal of Continuing Education in the Health Professions*, *26*(1), 13–24. https://doi.org/10.1002/chp.47

Greenhalgh, T., Robert, G., Macfarlane, F., Bate, P., & Kyriakidou, O. (2004). Diffusion of innovations in service organizations: systematic review and recommendations. *The Milbank Quarterly.* 82. 581–629. https://doi.org/10.1111/j.0887-378X.2004.00325.x

Kuiper, R. A., & Pesut, D. J. (2004). Promoting cognitive and metacognitive reflective reasoning skills in nursing practice: self-regulated learning theory. *Journal of Advanced Nursing, 45*(4): 381–391.

Langley, G. L., Moen, R., Nolan, K. M., Nolan, T. W., Norman, C. L., & Provost, L. P. (2009). *The improvement guide: A practical approach to enhancing organizational performance* (2nd ed.). Jossey-Bass Publishers.

McGlynn, E. A. (1998). Choosing and evaluating clinical performance measures. *Joint Commission Journal of Quality Improvement*, *24*(9), 470–479. https://doi.org/10.1016/s1070-3241(16)30396-0

Newhouse, R. P., Dearholt, S., Poe, S., Pugh, L. C., & White, K. M. (2007). Organizational change strategies for evidence-based practice. *JONA: The Journal of Nursing Administration*, *37*(12), 552–557. https://doi.org/10.1097/01.NNA.0000302384.91366.8f

Newhouse, R. P., & White, K. M. (2011). Guiding implementation: Frameworks and resources for evidence translation. *JONA: The Journal of Nursing Administration*, *41*(12), 513–516. https://doi.org/0.1097/NNA.0b013e3182378bb0

Nieva, V. F., Murphy, R., Ridley, N., Donaldson, N., Combes, J., Mitchell, P., Kovner, C., Hoy, E., & Carpenter, D. (2005). From science to service: A framework for the transfer of patient safety research into practice. *Advances in Patient Safety: From Research to Implementation* (Volume 2: Concepts and Methodology).

Poe, S., & White, K. (Eds.). (2010). *Johns Hopkins Nursing: Implementation and translation*. Sigma Theta Tau.

Pronovost, P. J., Miller, M. R., Dorman, T., Berenholtz, S. M., & Rubin, H. (2001). Developing and implementing measures of quality of care in the intensive care unit. *Current Opinion in Critical Care*, *7*(4), 297–303. https://doi.org/10.1097/00075198-200108000-00014

Schein, E. H. (2004). *Organizational culture and leadership* (3rd ed.). Jossey-Bass.

Stetler, C. B. (2001). Updating the Stetler Model of research utilization to facilitate evidence-based practice. *Nursing Outlook*, *49*(6), 272–279. https://doi.org/10.1067/mno.2001.120517

Stetler, C. B. (2010). Stetler Model. In J. Rycroft-Malone & T. Bucknall (Eds.), *Models and frameworks for implementing evidence-based practice: Linking evidence to action*. Wiley-Blackwell.

Stetler, C. B., Mittman, B. S., & Francis, J. (2008). Overview of the VA Quality Enhancement Research Initiative (QUERI) and QUERI theme articles: QUERI series. *Implementation Science*, *3*(1), 8. https://doi.org/10.1186/1748-5908-3-8

Tabak, R. G., Khoong, E. C., Chambers, D. A., & Brownson, R. C. (2012). Bridging research and practice: Models for dissemination and implementation research. *American Journal of Preventive Medicine*, *43*(3), 337–350. https://doi.org/10.1016/j.amepre.2012.05.024

Victor-Chmil, J. (2013). Critical thinking versus clinical reasoning versus clinical judgment: Differential diagnosis. *Nurse Educator*, *38*(1), 34–36. https://doi.org/10.1097/NNE.0b013e318276dfbe

Waltz, T. J., Powell, B. J., Matthieu, M. M., Damschroder, L. J., Chinman, M. J., Smith, J. L., Proctor, E. K., & Kirchner, J. E. (2015). Use of concept mapping to characterize relationships among implementation strategies and assess their feasibility and importance: Results from the Expert Recommendations for Implementing Change (ERIC) study. *Implementation Science*, *10*, 109. https://doi.org/10.1186/s13012-015-0295-0

White, K. M., Dudley-Brown, S., & Terhaar, M. (2020). *Translation of evidence into nursing and health care practice* (2nd ed.). Springer Publishing.

Dissemination

The final step of an EBP project is dissemination. Dissemination is an explicit process to share knowledge with a target audience to influence process or practice changes (Agency for Healthcare Research and Quality [AHRQ], 2014; Wilson, 2010). According to Serrat (2017) "at the simplest level, dissemination is best described as the delivery and receipt of a message, the engagement of an individual in a process, or the transfer of a process or product. Dissemination serves three broadly different purposes: awareness, understanding, and action" (p. 872). While completing an EBP project may have direct benefits to the EBP team's setting, successful dissemination can serve as the basis for evidence-based changes on a much broader scale. Formulating and following a dissemination plan, both within the team's organization and to an external audience, can ensure the highest impact of an EBP project.

This chapter explains the process of dissemination of an EBP project and provides examples of various strategies. The objectives are to describe:

- The process of creating a dissemination plan
- Internal and external dissemination options
- Audience-specific strategies for internal dissemination
- External conference presentations and publications
- Details, including strengths and weaknesses, of various dissemination strategies

How to Create a Dissemination Plan

Creating a purposeful dissemination plan helps to ensure the findings of an EBP project result in impactful changes. When developing a plan, the team should consider the following elements: the purpose of the dissemination, the message to be disseminated, the audience, the timing, and the method (AHRQ, 2014).

- **Purpose:** The purpose for dissemination will drive all other factors and can include raising awareness, informing, and promoting results (AHRQ, 2014).
- **Message:** Messages should be clear, targeted, actionable, and repeated (AHRQ, 2014; Scala, 2019).
- **Audience:** Previously identified stakeholders should inform decisions about the intended audience. While the overall purpose is the same, tailoring the message will depend on the intended recipients and their interests. Teams should adjust messaging accordingly (AHRQ, 2014).
- **Timing:** Timing can also be an important consideration and varies by stakeholders. For example, the start of the fiscal year might be an appropriate time to target leadership, or policy renewal windows may be a prime time to influence standards of practice. Additionally, topics can fall in and out of popularity, and the EBP team can capitalize on a focus from legislators or professional nursing organizations. Messages should

also be repeated. The "Marketing Rule of 7" suggests it may take up to seven contacts for a person to take a desired action (Goncalves, 2017).

- **Method:** There are numerous approaches to sharing information, from a staff email to a peer-reviewed publication. The method should match the intended reach of the message and be tailored to the specific audience. To reach the most people, the same idea should be spread through a variety of channels (AHRQ, 2014; Scala, 2019).

Internal Dissemination

It is important to share the results of the team's EBP project within their organization and within the specific setting and population indicated in the PICO question. Dissemination within the organization starts with the development of an effective communication plan specific to the internal audiences. This plan should ensure messaging occurs through multiple channels, is timely and frequent, is quickly and easily digestible, is personalized to the audience, is benefit focused, and solicits action (Scala, 2019).

Communication Strategies for Hospital Units/Departments

Once they determine the purpose of the dissemination, the EBP project team needs to identify existing communication strategies within their organization. Standard communication venues include newsletters, internal websites, private social media groups, journal clubs, grand rounds, staff meetings, and unit-based in-services. More customized communication strategies might include simulation scenarios, development of pocket cards, tool kits, focus groups, podcasts, or lunch-and-learns. Once the team identifies the communication venues and strategies that are available to them, they need to identify the how, what, and format of the information to be shared. A key strategy is to ensure that each piece of communication to internal stakeholders has a focus of answering the question of "what's in it for the staff?" (Scala, 2019). This will ensure the communication lets staff know specifically what will change for them and what role they will have in the change.

Communication Strategies for Executive Leadership

An *executive summary* is a written method of dissemination used to present the outcomes of the project within the organization at the executive or director level. An executive summary is typically a one- to two-page document that includes:

- Description of the current state of the problem within the organization/setting
- Why the change is needed
- Overview of the project that outlines how the project aligns with the strategic priorities and mission/vision of the organization
- Implementation process
- Evaluation metrics
- Project outcomes as they relate to specific metrics:
    - Financial
    - Patient satisfaction
    - Clinical
    - Other
- Sustainability plan
- Other organizational implications

Challenges Related to Internal Dissemination

Evidence-based practice projects can spark small or large changes in an organization. These may be met with predictable or even unexpected challenges, and an effective internal dissemination plan is a powerful strategy to move forward with the team's desired change. Refer to Chapter 2 for a review of the stages of change versus transition. Understanding change management strategies helps determine the best type of messaging depending on the emotional components of the project's recommendations.

External Dissemination

There are many ways to share the results of an EBP project with an audience outside of the EBP team's organization. Because the EBP process involves many steps, the team has several opportunities to share the project throughout its life cycle. This type of dissemination does not always follow a set path, but typically, projects move from conference presentation to manuscript publication. The following sections review methods for external dissemination.

Conferences

Generally, professional organizations host scientific conferences that act as a platform for learning and networking. They can take place at the local, state, regional, national, and international levels. To provide relevant content, conference organizers typically solicit applications for poster or podium presentations to take place during the event. Most conferences have themes, and depending on the size, may have specific categories or tracks for content. For example, the American Nurses Credentialing Center (ANCC) National Magnet Conference 2019 theme was "Educate. Innovate. Celebrate." with tracks such as evidence-based practice, leadership, innovation, and research (2019). Each conference is unique in its requirements, but the center of most calls for presentation submissions is an abstract. This provides a short, high-level summary to the organizers to guide their decision on both the quality and the fit of the content for their program. When planning to submit to a conference, presenters should reference the event website, which usually provides details on the specific elements required (e.g., references, objectives, relevance to the field). Visit your profession's general and specialty organization websites for potential conference opportunities.

Poster presentations can be a physical printout or a digital display of a team's work. The benefits of these presentations are they can be easy to read, encourage networking with colleagues, and have a much quicker turn-around time than writing and editing a manuscript (Edwards, 2015; Serrat, 2017). One major drawback is to the abbreviated nature of the content because it is difficult to convey the depth and rigor of a project in a 3 × 4-foot visual display. Conferences can also be costly to attend (Edwards, 2015; Serrat, 2017). When designing a poster, here are some tips to keep in mind:

- Templates are often available to guide the design. The team's organization or the conference may provide blank prototypes in PowerPoint for the authors to customize with their project information.
- Pictures, figures, and graphs make data not only visually appealing, but also digestible. When possible, consider displaying information as an image.
- Most people will be reading a poster from several feet away. Make sure all content is readable at that distance. For reference, on a printed 3 × 4 foot poster, 40-point font will stand 1 inch tall.
- While the inclination can be to share as much information as possible, white space is very important and can make a poster much more visually appealing as well as readable for someone passing by.

Podium presentations give the presenter an opportunity to share their work in an oral format, usually with slides as a visual aid. Presentation formats include individual presenters, teams, or groups of panelists. Podium presentations have the advantages of being engaging for the audience, allowing time for in-depth explanation as well as question and answer sessions. On the downside, they were typically only available to those in attendance; however, the abundance of virtual events since the COVID-19 pandemic has extended their reach. Additionally, the effectiveness of the presentation can rely heavily on the skills of the presenters (Foulkes, 2015; Serrat, 2017). Tips on creating and delivering an effective and engaging podium presentation are:

- While putting together the presentation, determine a clear message and strategy to convey that message to the specific audience (Reynolds, 2010).
- People can read or they can listen; it is hard to do both. Use text sparingly and in short phrases (Duarte, 2008; Foulkes, 2015).

- Slides should serve as an outline, or talking points, not a script. Do not read directly from the slides. A good rule is that the presenter should still be able to give the presentation even if the equipment fails (Duarte, 2008; Foulkes, 2015; Reynolds, 2010).
- Graphics and pictures can be helpful but should not take away from the content. Be wary of using animations or bright or clashing colors because these can be distracting (Duarte, 2008; Foulkes, 2015).
- When using colored text or backgrounds, ensure all text is easily readable and in a legible font from a distance. Keep in mind that color slides may be printed in grayscale. Fonts should be consistent across all slides unless used for emphasis (Duarte, 2008).

Peer-Reviewed Journal Articles

Not only is the EBP process dependent on the availability of scientific literature, the completion of an EBP project has the potential to add to the available knowledge on a topic through the peer-reviewed publication process. While the publication process can be time-intensive, it has the benefits of being a well-established and thorough method to ensure the information being shared meets the standards of the journal and by extension the scientific community. Once published, the information shared in the article is not limited to people in attendance at a conference and can have a wide reach (Serrat, 2017). Figure 9.1 represents an overview of the typical article publication process. Other important elements when preparing a manuscript include identifying an appropriate target journal as well as adhering to the relevant publication standards and reporting guidelines.

Selecting a suitable journal for a manuscript submission involves several factors. The process begins by reviewing the journal's website to determine the types of submissions they accept and their target audience. Additionally, reviewing recent publications will provide insights into the journal's areas of interest. The EBP team's submission should be a good fit for the scope of the journal but also fill a gap in their published content. For example, if the journal recently published an article on a very similar topic, they may be more reticent to publish duplicative material. Other factors to consider are the journal's acceptance rate and *impact factor* (a calculation often used as an indicator of reach or importance of the journal; Lariviere & Sugimoto, 2019). In the early stages of the publication process, the EBP team can also query a journal's editor to gauge interest in a potential submission. This might provide important feedback that would not be gleaned from the webpage alone.

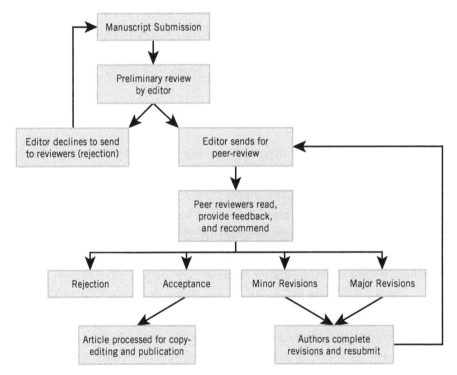

Figure 9.1 Manuscript pathway from submission to publication.

To find potential journals, websites such as the International Academy of Nursing Editors' (INANE) page (https://nursingeditors.com/), the Journal/Author Name Estimator (https://jane.biosemantics.org/), and InCites Journal Citation Reports (https://jcr.clarivate.com) can provide useful information. Additionally, many professional healthcare organizations have an associated journal that may be a good fit in the team's given field. Finally, the authors should be aware of predatory publishing. There is no standardized definition of "predatory journal," but the term includes characteristics such as deceptiveness or lack of transparency, unethical practices, persuasive language, poor quality standards, and large or hidden article processing fees (Cobey et al., 2018; McLeod et al., 2018). Resources on how to identify and avoid these journals reside on Beall's list (https://beallslist.net/). See Box 9.1 for information on citing authorship.

> **Box 9.1 Citing Authorship**
>
> Authorship is an important part of external dissemination. According to the International Committee of Medical Journal Editors (2021), authorship should be based on four criteria:
>
> - Substantial contributions to the conception or design of the work; or the acquisition, analysis, or interpretation of data for the work; AND
> - Drafting the work or revising it critically for important intellectual content; AND
> - Final approval of the version to be published; AND
> - Agreement to be accountable for all aspects of the work in ensuring that questions related to the accuracy or integrity of any part of the work are appropriately investigated and resolved.
>
> It is important to establish an authorship plan and expectations at the beginning of a project. Further guidance can be found at http://www.icmje.org/recommendations/browse/roles-and-responsibilities/.

After selecting a target journal, it is important to review the author instructions carefully. There the team will find specific requirements for the journal as well as reference to publication standards and reporting guidelines. A reporting guideline is a simple, structured tool for the team to use while writing manuscripts and includes a "checklist, flow diagram, or structured text to guide authors in reporting a specific type of research, developed using explicit methodology" (EQUATOR Network). The appropriate standards depend on the type of project (e.g., quality improvement, randomized control trial, systematic reviews), but all manuscripts will include some basic elements displayed in Table 9.1. (For writing tips, see Box 9.2.) A list of reporting standards can be found on the Enhancing the QUAlity and Transparency Of health Research (EQUATOR) Network website (https://www.equator-network.org/contact/contact/). As of 2020, there are no widely established reporting standards for EBP projects. Based on EBP quality guidelines, as well as recommendations for reporting by the Cochrane Review and JBI, this text includes a writing template for Publishing on Evidence-Based Practice Projects (see Appendix J).

Table 9.1 Components of a Manuscript Submission

Parts of a Manuscript Submission	Description
Cover Letter	A letter written to the publisher of a journal briefly describing the intent of the submission and why it is of interest to the journal.
Title Page	A separate document that contains the names, affiliations, and credentials of the authors to maintain anonymity in the manuscript itself.
Introduction	A brief description of the problem, available knowledge on the subject, and the question the study is attempting to address.
Methods	A description of the design of the study, including what was done and how it was evaluated. This section should read as a guide or manual on the process.
Results	An overall description of the major findings and the data itself. The results section does not include commentary or discussion, just facts and figures.
Discussion	A summary of findings and how the findings compare to the current state of the science on the topic. It also should include any limitations, implications, or future directions of the work.

Hall, 2012

Other Types of Dissemination

While conference presentations and peer-reviewed manuscripts are the most traditional external dissemination routes, there are other avenues to share scientific knowledge. These can still include publication-based pieces such as articles in professional journals or magazines (non-peer-reviewed), book chapters, opinion pieces, interviews, video abstracts, and letters to the editor. Additionally, more social media–based alternatives such as blogs, Twitter, Facebook, and YouTube are becoming ever more popular and may be able to reach a broader audience (Gates et al., 2018; Hoang et al., 2015; Konkiel et al., 2016; Markham et al., 2017; Scala, 2019). These alternative types of dissemination may be a good starting point for people new to the scientific writing process. Additionally, research shows evidence-based practices have slow and incomplete uptake. Engaging in alternate forms of dissemination is one approach to ensure information reaches clinicians and patients (Gates et al., 2018; Gregory & Twells, 2015).

> **Box 9.2 Hints for Writing**
> - When writing a manuscript, write the abstract last. When preparing a poster or podium presentation, write the abstract first.
> - You can only submit to one journal at a time.
> - For conferences, scoring rubrics are usually used to determine a certain number per track, not total, so some tracks may be less competitive than others.
> - For online conference submissions, write (and save) the submission in a separate document first. Many online submission systems do not have word counters, spell check, etc.
> - Conferences can solicit submissions sometimes up to a year in advance, so be sure to keep an eye on anything of interest.
>
> More writing resources can be found at http://oedb.org/ilibrarian/150-writing-resources.

Summary

Dissemination of EBP projects can take various forms and is an essential step in the EBP process. As members of the healthcare community, the EBP team has the opportunity to improve the accessibility of knowledge to enhance the state of the science on a given topic and catalyze change. The importance of dissemination cannot be discounted and has even been included in healthcare providers' Codes of Ethics, including the American Nurses Association (ANA) and the American Medical Association (AMA). These documents call for the advancement of the profession through various scientific approaches, including research development, evaluation, prompt dissemination, and application to practice (AMA, 2016; ANA, 2015). Clinically practicing healthcare professionals completing an EBP project are in the unique position to provide firsthand knowledge of patient care coupled with best practice evidence and realistic recommendations. Dissemination is a tool to advocate for patients, staff, and populations and is an opportunity for the EBP team to promote the science and healthcare professions.

References

Agency for Healthcare Research and Quality. (2014). *Quick-start guide to dissemination for practice-based research networks*. https://pbrn.ahrq.gov/sites/default/files/AHRQ%20PBRN%20Dissemination%20QuickStart%20Guide_0.pdf

American Medical Association. (2016). AMA principles of medical ethics. https://www.ama-assn.org/delivering-care/ama-principles-medical-ethics

American Nurses Association (2015). *Code of ethics for nurses with interpretative statements*. Author.

ANCC National Magnet Conference. (2019). https://ancc.confex.com/ancc/f/ixqzozlktzwq

Cobey, K. D., Lalu, M. M., Skidmore, B., Ahmadzai, N., Grudniewicz, A., & Moher, D. (2018). What is a predatory journal? A scoping review. *F1000Research*, 7. https://doi.org/10.12688/f1000research.15256.2

Duarte, N. (2008). *Slide: ology: The art and science of creating great presentations* (Vol. 1). O'Reilly Media.

Edwards, D. J. (2015). Dissemination of research results: On the path to practice change. *The Canadian Journal of Hospital Pharmacy*, 68(6), 465–469. https://doi.org/10.4212/cjhp.v68i6.1503

EQUATOR Network. (n.d.). Centre for Statistics in Medicine, Nuffield Department of Orthopaedics, Rheumatology and Musculoskeletal Sciences (NDORMS), University of Oxford. https://www.equator-network.org/contact/contact/

Foulkes, M. (2015). Presentation skills for nurses. *Nursing Standard (2014+)*, 29(25), 52.

Gates, A., Featherstone, R., Shave, K., Scott, S. D., & Hartling, L. (2018). Dissemination of evidence in paediatric emergency medicine: A quantitative descriptive evaluation of a 16-week social media promotion. *BMJ Open*, 8(6), e022298. https://doi.org/10.1136/bmjopen-2018-022298

Goncalves, P. (2017). *Want successful employee communications? Think like a marketer*. Strategic HR Review.

Gregory, D. M., & Twells, L. K. (2015). Evidence-based decision-making 5: Translational research. In P. S. Parfrey & B. J. Barrett (Eds.), *Clinical epidemiology* (pp. 455–468). Humana Press.

Hall, G. M. (Ed.). (2012). *How to write a paper*. John Wiley & Sons.

Hoang, J. K., McCall, J., Dixon, A. F., Fitzgerald, R. T., & Gaillard, F. (2015). Using social media to share your radiology research: how effective is a blog post? *Journal of the American College of Radiology*, 12(7), 760–765. https://doi.org/10.1016/j.jacr.2015.03.048

International Committee of Medical Journal Editors. 2021. [cited 2014 Apr 14]. *Roles and responsibilities of authors, contributors, reviewers, editors, publishers, and owners: Protection of Research Participants.*

Konkiel, S., Madjarevic, N., & Rees, A. (2016). *Altmetrics for librarians: 100+ tips, tricks, and examples: Brought to you by Altmetric*. Altmetric LLP.

Lariviere, V., & Sugimoto, C. R. (2019). The journal impact factor: A brief history, critique, and discussion of adverse effects. In W. Glänzel, H. F. Moed, U. Schmoch, & M. Thelwall (Eds.), *Springer handbook of science and technology indicators* (pp. 3–24). Springer.

Lee, M. C., Johnson, K. L., Newhouse, R. P., & Warren, J. I. (2013). Evidence-based practice process quality assessment: EPQA guidelines. *Worldviews on Evidence Based Nursing*, 10(3), 140–149. https://doi.org/10.1111/j.1741-6787.2012.00264.x

Markham, M. J., Gentile, D., & Graham, D. L. (2017). Social media for networking, professional development, and patient engagement. *American Society of Clinical Oncology Educational Book*, 37, 782–787. https://doi.org/10.1200/EDBK_180077

McLeod, A., Savage, A., & Simkin, M. G. (2018). The ethics of predatory journals. *Journal of Business Ethics*, 153(1), 121–131. https://doi.org/10.1007/s10551-016-3419-9

Reynolds, G. (2010). *The naked presenter: Delivering powerful presentations with or without slides*. Pearson Education.

Scala, E., Whalen, M., Parks, J., Ascenzi, J., & Pandian, V. (2019). Increasing nursing research program visibility: A systematic review and implementation of the evidence. *JONA: The Journal of Nursing Administration*, 49(12), 617–623.

Serrat, O. (2017). Disseminating knowledge products. In O. Serrat (Ed.), *Knowledge solutions* (pp. 871–878). Springer.

Wilson, P. M., Petticrew, M., Calnan, M. W., & Nazareth, I. (2010). Disseminating research findings: What should researchers do? A systematic scoping review of conceptual frameworks. *Implementation Science*, 5(1), 91.

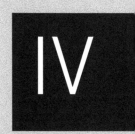

Exemplars

10 Exemplars............................223

10

Exemplars

Learning While Going Through the Process of an Evidence-Based Practice Project

Nancy M. Beck MSN, RN, NDP-BC
Jackie Bradstock BSN, RN, PCCN
The Johns Hopkins Hospital, Baltimore, MD, USA

Practice Question

At The Johns Hopkins Hospital (JHH), policies and protocols require renewal every three years, necessitating review of the most recent evidence. A team of clinical nurses, clinical nurse specialists, and educators who sit on JHH's Department of Surgery standards of care committee reviewed the chest tube policy. Through conversation, the team discovered that practices as well as level of comfort when caring for a patient with chest tubes varied between units and departments.

After identifying these discrepancies, the committee decided they would use this opportunity to complete their first EBP project using the JHEBP model.

The team developed the background EBP question:

> *What are the best practices for nursing management and care of chest tubes (I) in the in-patient setting (P)?*

Evidence

The EBP team completed a review of the literature using numerous search terms (e.g., *chest tubes, dressings*) in PubMed and CINAHL. The medical librarian at JHH was essential in completing this literature search. Keywords searched included *chest tube, placement, insertion, removal, pain, pain management, dressing, occlusive dressing, securement, stripping, milking, suction, drainage, assessment, education, best practice, guidelines,* and *policies.* Inclusion criteria included English language journal, adult patients, and publication within the last 10 years. The articles underwent a title, abstract, and full text screening for relevance to the practice question by two individual reviewers. The group organized the results using specific categories. Initially the research yielded 173 articles. Of these articles, 31 met inclusion criteria. The team appraised those 31 articles for level and quality using the JHEBP model; see Figure 10.1.

The evidence entailed six random control trials (RCT), 11 clinical practice guidelines, and three quality improvement (QI) projects, with the remainder being quasi-experimental, systematic reviews, prospective descriptive, and quantitative designs. Overall, synthesis of the evidence revealed a lack of compelling evidence to make drastic changes to the protocol. Our current practice for accidental tube removal was consistent with the literature. The evidence did not indicate a superior method for tube-to-tube securement or chest tube dressing. Several articles supported digital over analog drainage systems. Evidence also indicated that delivering education to nurses by self-learning modules was effective, and the use of a bedside checklist might prevent adverse events. Regarding pain, cold therapy was determined to be effective. Other evidence supported our current practice of intermittent clamping and discouraged milking and stripping.

Level	Quantity	Quality
Level 1	5	A–B
Level 2	4	A–B
Level 3	5	B
Level 4	11	A–B
Level 5	6	A–B

Figure 10.1　Articles appraised, listed by level and quality.

Translation

Due to the lack of compelling evidence, the team recommended only minor changes to the management of patients with chest tubes protocol. Because there is high-quality Level I evidence supporting the use of cold therapy for pain management and the goal of improving comfort levels related to caring for patients with chest tubes, the team added this to the policy under the "care management" section. With the goal of improving comfort levels related to caring for patients with chest tubes, the team also added a new appendix containing a bedside checklist based on the evidence findings. Advancing the state of the science on dressings, tube-to-tube securement, and digital versus analog systems requires more research.

Outcomes

One of the biggest outcomes of this policy review EBP project was exposing staff to evidence-based practice and the JHNEBP model. People with no previous exposure to EBP were able to practice the process from start to finish. It was a valuable and enjoyable learning experience. Although the evidence did not indicate major policy changes, the EBP project validated our current practices, such as those for accidental tube removal, chest tube dressings, and tube-to-tube securement. Nurse educators within the department created online modules to train nurses in the care and management of chest tubes. Additionally, didactic and experiential classes allow nurses additional opportunity for learning and practice. Finally, the educators distributed the bedside checklist to all nursing staff. Nurses readily endorsed the increased educational opportunities and checklist guidance during informal discussions. Next steps include creating an online module about the care and management of patients with chest tubes for initial and on-going education for all nurses. In addition, the team will continue to watch for new evidence regarding topics such as dressings, tube-to-tube securement, and use of digital versus analog systems that may address the EBP question.

Prevention of LVAD Driveline Infections

Tania Randell, MS, RN, ACCNS-AG
Tim Madeira, MS, RN, ACNP-BC, CCNS, CCRN, PCCN
Martha Abshire, PhD, RN
The Johns Hopkins Hospital, Baltimore, MD, USA

Practice Question

Implantation of a left ventricular assist device (LVAD) is a life-prolonging surgical therapy for people suffering from end-stage heart failure. The LVAD circulates blood from the left ventricle, through a pump, returning it to the aorta, therefore improving cardiac output. Power to the LVAD is supplied through a driveline (DL) exiting the patient's abdomen. However, among hospitals across the nation, care of the driveline remains varied and not standardized. Care of the driveline by staff, patients, and caregivers is a key component in preventing infections and subsequent complications such as bleeding, pain, antibiotic resistance, thrombosis, and stroke.

After noting multiple patient readmissions due to driveline infection (DLI), Clinical Nurse Specialists from two cardiac units formed a collaborative team to address the problem of driveline infection within The Johns Hopkins Hospital System (JHHS). At the inception of the project, DLI rates at JHHS were well above the national benchmark, making it imperative to search the literature for best practices. To examine the available literature and develop an evidence-based solution, an EBP question was created to guide the literature search and frame the project:

> *In adult LVAD patients (P), how do driveline dressing change strategies (I) compared to standard care (C) affect the incidence of driveline infections (O) during the first year of post-operative recovery?*

Evidence

The team conducted an advanced literature search using the PubMed, CINAHL, and Embase databases. Keyword search terms were combined using Boolean connectors and included the words *"left ventricular assist device" "OR" "LVAD" "OR" "mechanical circulatory support" "OR" "MCS" "AND" "infection" "OR" "infect*" "AND" "driveline"*. To refine the initial 1,143 search results, the team constructed a PRISMA diagram. Inclusion criteria limited articles to research, clinical trials, randomized controlled trials, observational studies, systematic reviews, meta-analysis, peer-reviewed, full text, and English language. Sixteen articles remained, yet only five titles matched the PICO question. The final review included one Level II systematic review, three Level III research studies, and one Level IV clinical practice guideline. The EBP team critically appraised and rated the five studies to determine evidence level and quality using the JH-NEBP Model Evidence Appraisal tools. One article received a quality rating of A, and the remaining four articles received a quality rating of B; thus, the evidence synthesis indicated good-quality evidence. Four of the five articles found that dressing change protocols significantly reduced the incidence of driveline infections. The remaining article found that a dressing change protocol was associated with an overall reduction in 30-day readmission rates but was not statistically significant. Evidence suggested that there is moderate-to-substantial certainty that a driveline dressing change bundle is beneficial to the prevention of DLI.

Translation

Based on these results and general best practices in patient care and infection prevention, we began a quality improvement (QI) project using the Plan-Do-Study-Act (PDSA) methodology. Implementation of the DLI QI project consisted of six key elements:

- Standardize practices through the creation of a driveline dressing change kit
- Update policies related to driveline dressing care
- Select and train nursing unit champions
- Educate all nursing staff across the five JHHS units caring for LVAD patients
- Educate patients and caregivers using an instructional video and in-person demonstration
- Develop strategies and tactics to ensure practice change sustainment

The team collected initial pre- and post-implementation data over a four-year period, spanning 2016–2020, with the intervention occurring in late 2018. The number of new infections during the first post-operative year declined to 3 infections from 11 infections pre-intervention, although not statistically significant (Fisher's Exact, p=0.078). The overall rate declined from 33.3% to 12.5% in one year and is currently zero percent for calendar year 2020. Dissemination of the project findings included internally as a report to the Quality Assurance Performance Improvement (QAPI) committee and externally as a poster presentation to the Heart Failure Society of America (HFSA).

Summary

Prior to implementation of this DLI QI project, DLI rates at JHHS were more than double the national benchmark. Two years post implementation, the DLI rates at JHHS have declined below the benchmark. Improvement in the DLI rate was achievable only after description of the problem, creation of an EBP question, systematic literature review, implementation of a quality improvement initiative, and multiple iterations of the PDSA cycle. Promotion of ongoing quality improvement and sustainability through implementation of the evidence requires continued research.

Outpatient Palliative Care to Improve Quality of Life and Reduce Symptom Burden and 30-Day Readmissions in Patients With Heart Failure

Kelly Trynosky, DNP, RN, ACNP-BC Wellspan Ephrata Hospital, Ephrata, PA, USA

Practice Question

Heart failure (HF) is a devastating chronic illness affecting over 6.5 million Americans. Each year, 960,000 new cases emerge, with an expected prevalence of over 8 million cases in this country by 2030. HF is a debilitating disease with significant burden on patients, families, and the healthcare system. Patients with HF often have distressing symptoms requiring hospitalization for treatment. Across the disease trajectory, the symptoms associated with HF progress, causing a significant decline in quality of life (QOL). The progressive nature of HF not only affects patients but also their caregivers by causing increased stress as it becomes more and more difficult to care for them at home. Managing the symptoms of HF to improve QOL and prevent hospitalizations is imperative.

Palliative care is a specialized field of medicine that works collaboratively with the patient's existing providers, focusing on managing symptoms and reducing suffering. The topic of palliative care typically arises in the inpatient setting when patients and families are experiencing emergent situations and burden of illness. This may leave little time to address important goals of care, including long-term symptom management. The goals of palliative care involvement, such as to improve symptom burden, discuss advanced care planning, and offer support for patients and families, may be best served in the outpatient setting with longitudinal support. Despite recommendations in the scientific literature, there is limited use of palliative care in the outpatient setting for HF patients. This evidence-based project investigated the question:

> *In patients with HF (P), does the delivery of palliative care in the outpatient clinic (I) improve quality of life and reduce symptom burden and 30-day readmissions (O) compared to standard heart failure care (C)?*

Evidence

This question guided an online literature search using the databases of PubMed, Ovid, and Google Scholar. The search was limited to publication years 2008–2018 with terms including *palliative medicine, palliative care, heart failure, outpatient, ambulatory*, and *palliative nursing*. The initial search identified 41 articles. Relevant articles included those relating to outpatient palliative care with outcomes including symptom management and QOL, with priority given to articles specifically identifying team-oriented care between palliative care and HF teams. Further review focused on articles relating to outpatient palliative care involvement, evaluation of QOL, and coordination of care with HF teams, yielding 13 articles for appraisal. Due to limited evidence with readmission outcomes, a second search was conducted using the same databases and publication dates with search terms *palliative care, heart failure*, and *readmissions*. This search identified an additional 27 articles, with two articles relevant to outpatient care and readmission outcomes yielding 15 articles for appraisal; see Figure 10.2. The synthesized scientific evidence supported further integration of outpatient palliative care in the care of the HF population.

Level	# Articles	Quality
I	3	B
II	4	B
III	6	B
IV	1	A
V	1	B

Figure 10.2 The found articles, listed by level and quality.

Translation

Implementation included providing palliative care services to adult HF patients in an existing outpatient HF disease management program over a 12-week period. Participants received an initial consult with a palliative care team including a nurse practitioner and social worker, with subsequent follow-up visits at weeks

4 and 8. Assessments at baseline and weeks 4 and 8 explored QOL (Kansas City Cardiomyopathy Questionnaire) and symptom burden (Edmonton Symptom Assessment Scale). Mean QOL and symptom burden scores improved from 48.44 to 66.67 ($p = 0.867$) and 24 to 21 ($p = 0.317$), respectively, over the 12-week intervention period. Although the project offered no statistically significant findings regarding readmission rates, hospitalizations were fewer after palliative care than before. Those with two or more hospitalizations prior to palliative care intervention had a 71.4% decrease post intervention ($p = 0.59$).

Summary

The findings from this evidence-based project were consistent with existing scientific research, demonstrating how outpatient palliative care complements standard HF care and can improve quality of life and reduce symptom burden in patients with HF. The clinical significance of the outcomes offers noteworthy opportunities for healthcare systems to avoid hospitalizations and readmission penalties. Misconceptions of the purpose of palliative care by providers, patients, and families proved to be the largest barrier during implementation. Ongoing education through dissemination of these findings includes the system, state, and national levels to bridge this gap. Delivery of palliative care in the outpatient HF clinic provides an innovative approach to this high-risk population. Palliative care is an integral part of the HF disease management team and has the potential to be the differentiator in best practice models of HF care.

Implementation of a Saline and Pulsatile Flush Procedure for Central Venous Catheters

MiKaela Olsen DNP, APRN-CNS, AOCNS, FAAN
The Johns Hopkins Hospital, Baltimore, MD, USA

Practice Question

Management of cancer patients undergoing complex therapies—including blood products, parenteral nutrition, electrolyte replacement, and chemotherapy—often requires central venous access catheters (CVCs). An anticoagulant, heparin, used as a flush solution for maintenance of catheter patency, has been the standard for decades. The practice of flushing heparin into peripheral intravenous and arterial catheters halted in the 1990s when landmark studies demonstrated no difference in occlusions between saline and heparin flushes.

Although heparin can increase the risk of serious patient harm and cost, healthcare providers are reluctant to use a saline-only flush solution in cancer patients with CVCs due to a concern for increased thrombotic occlusions. Associated with serious complications, heparin can cause bleeding, allergic reactions, stimulation of biofilm formation in many strains of S. aureus, coagulase-negative staphylococci, and heparin-induced thrombocytopenia (HIT). Biofilm may shield bacteria from antibiotics, increasing the risk of antibiotic failure. HIT prevalence ranges from 0.1% to 5% in patients receiving heparin. This complication can occur after minimal heparin exposure, including heparin flush, and has been associated with serious outcomes such as thrombosis, bleeding, and death. Given the risks of heparin, this Clinical Nurse Specialist (CNS) initiated an evidence-based practice project to determine whether a safer flush alternative was feasible.

Evidence

The purpose of this EBP project was to determine whether saline flush using a pulsatile or turbulent technique could maintain central venous catheters in adult oncology patients instead of heparin. PICO question:

> *In adult patients with cancer who have central venous access devices (P), how does saline using a pulsatile flush technique (I) compared to heparin flush (C) affect thrombotic catheter occlusion (O)?*

Johns Hopkins Welch Library, MEDLINE, and CINAHL were the databases used for the literature search. Keywords included: *central venous catheters, central venous catheter, central vascular catheter, central vascular catheters, central vascular lines, saline, sodium chloride, NaCl, lock, flush, flushing, neoplasms, neoplasm, cancer, cancers, leukemia, lymphoma, sarcoma, carcinoma, occlusion, occlusions*. Inclusion criteria was limited to English-language, peer-reviewed articles. Articles were excluded that were older than six years. Studies included oncology patients with central vascular access devices. For this EBP review, 24 articles were included. Fifteen randomized controlled trials have been included in four systematic reviews and one meta-analysis for this EBP project. Each individual study received a quality rating using the JHNEBP Quality Rating scheme for Research Evidence. Of the 15 RCT Level I studies, 11 provided high-quality (A) results showing no significant difference between heparin and saline flush for CVCs, and 4 provided good (B) quality results. Four systematic reviews and one meta-analysis were graded as high (A) quality. Three additional articles included two retrospective observational cohort studies and a consensus guideline, graded at high (A) or good (B) quality. The two retrospective studies also demonstrated no difference between the two flushes with regard to CVC occlusions. The consensus guideline was graded using the Appraisal of Guidelines for Research and Evaluation (AGREE) II tool. These guidelines had an overall rating of 6.

Evidence synthesis concluded that:

- Heparin is not superior to normal saline for flushing CVCs.
- Heparin increases cost and the risk of patient harm (bleeding, infection, biofilm formation, heparin-induced thrombocytopenia).
- A pulsating flush procedure has been shown to be effective for reducing intraluminal buildup that can contributes to occlusions.
- Saline is an effective flush solution for CVCs in adult oncology patients when combined with a pulsatile flush procedure.

Translation

After review of the evidence, this DNP project lead conducted a focused education with a CVC flush skills lab, which significantly improved nursing staff compliance with a turbulent or pulsatile saline flush procedure and increased knowledge of the practice change. A saline and pulsatile flush protocol replaced heparin in November of 2018 at the practice setting. Patients with large bore catheters benefited the most from this practice change with the successful elimination of high doses of heparin to maintain catheter patency. The elimination of high dose heparin for flush in this patient population, who are at risk of bleeding due to thrombocytopenia and other serious complications, improved patient safety and decreased staff workload. The majority of patients did not require a de-clotting medication during the project-monitoring period, and the overall incidence of occlusion was similar to other published studies. Ongoing work will include the development of an algorithm for patients who develop occlusion. This will include reinforcement of the flush procedure for patients and caregivers, a more frequent saline flush routine, and assessment of proper catheter tip location to look for suboptimal placement.

This quality improvement project provides initial support regarding the feasibility of implementing a carefully designed saline and turbulent or pulsatile flush procedure for hematologic malignancy patients with CVCs. Saline and pulsatile flush is an effective and safe alternative to heparin for flushing of CVCs in hematologic malignancy patients.

At the time of this publication, the project practice site has surpassed the two-year mark with saline and pulsation flush for CVCs as standard of care. The entire Sidney Kimmel Comprehensive Cancer Center inpatient and outpatient went live with the saline and pulsatile flush protocol in January of 2020, with no significant increase in the number of occlusions observed. Future plans include implementation in adult, non-oncology patients at The Johns Hopkins Hospital and other Johns Hopkins affiliate sites.

Pressure Injury Prevention in the Surgical ICU

Susan Hammond, DNP, MBA, RN, NE-BC
Sarah Porter, MS, RN, NE-BC
Samantha Young, MS, RN, CCRN, ACNPC, CCNS
Susan Thul, DNP, APRN, CNM
Deborah Dang, PhD, RN, NEA-BC
The Johns Hopkins Hospital, Baltimore, MD, USA

Practice Question

Pressure injuries affect nearly 2.5 million hospitalized patients a year in the United States, leading to a financial cost of $9.1–$11.6 billion per year. Despite the fact pressure ulcers have been extensively studied and there is compelling evidence toward best practice, pressure injuries still exist and have significant negative impacts on the patient, their caregivers, and the healthcare system.

Patients in the intensive care unit (ICU) have a higher incidence of pressure injuries due to their level of acuity. Frequently, sedation, mechanical ventilation, hemodynamic instability, or trauma immobilizes these patients. Surgical ICUs (SICUs) have a higher incidence of hospital-acquired pressure injuries (HAPIs) compared to coronary care units.

The background PICO question driving this translational project is:

> *What are the best practices to prevent pressure ulcers (I/O) in an adult surgical intensive care unit (P)?*

Evidence

The team conducted a literature search to assess for current best practices in relation to pressure injuries in the adult surgical ICU population. The databases used to conduct the literature search included: PubMed/MEDLINE, CINAHL, and Google Scholar. The keywords included several Medical Subject Headings (MeSH): *pressure ulcer(s)*, *pressure injury(s)*, and *intensive care unit (ICU)* or *critical care*. The negative keywords, *pediatric* and *neonatal*, served to exclude results. The team excluded articles if they focused on care in nursing homes or subacute facilities. The search included only English-language articles and none older than 10 years, although the majority of the articles selected were less than five years old in order to maintain relevance to current practice. A final selection of 20 articles were included in a detailed review. The articles for the detailed appraisal described research from Argentina, Australia, Canada, Saudi Arabia, the United Kingdom, and the United States. Of the 20 articles, there were two Level II studies, both randomized control trials, with quality grades of high (A) or good (B). Both studies showed a reduction in pressure injuries with the implementation of a pressure injury prevention bundle. Five of the articles were Level III studies with either nonexperimental studies, systematic review of nonexperimental studies, or quasi-experimental studies, graded as A or B. All five articles suggested taking a multifaceted approach to implementing and sustaining an improvement, specifically pressure injury prevention bundles. Level IV (n=10) and Level V (n=3) reinforced that pressure injury prevention cannot be done successfully without taking a bundled, multidisciplinary approach. In summary, the articles indicated bundles are best practice, and interdisciplinary communication is imperative to improved patient outcomes.

Translation

Based on the evidence, a team reviewed current practice and the gaps in practice. The evidence-based interventions outlined a multifaceted approach for implementation in the SICU, including:

- The development of an evidence-based pressure injury prevention bundle decision tree, which reflected the hospital's pressure injury policy and wound care policy
- The use of theory-guided focus groups during pre-implementation to review the development of nursing in-services related to a pressure injury prevention decision tree
- The development of nursing in-services and voiceover PowerPoint related to the pressure injury prevention decision tree
- The development of a chart audit tracking tool to evaluate compliance with nursing documentation related to pressure injury prevention
- Monthly communication of results to frontline staff

The team established outcome goals of 90% compliance with the pressure injury documentation by six months post-implementation and incidence of pressure injuries in the WICU maintained below the national benchmark by six months post-implementation. The pre-implementation pressure injury prevention documentation compliance was 52% at six months post-implementation; pressure injury prevention documentation compliance was 76%, a 24% improvement. Overall, the pressure injury rates in the WICU showed improvement, but rates remained variable depending on the month and, potentially, the acuity level of the patients.

Summary

The implementation of this project led to overall improvement in the documentation compliance related to pressure injury prevention in the surgical ICU. The number of pressure injuries that developed post-implementation was lower than the pre-implementation months. However, when comparing the trend throughout the year, the results were variable, and one cannot conclude that this project implementation had a significant impact on pressure injury reduction in the WICU. Further statistical testing and analysis is required to determine the correlation between the implementation of this project and the reduction in pressure injuries in relation to the patient's acuity level.

Throughout this project, other changes within the unit also occurred that allowed for easier partnership with the wound care team and more education of the WICU staff on pressure injuries and prevention. The team disseminated the project findings on the institutional, local, and state level. Next steps include sharing the evidence-based decision tree with other units throughout the hospital and potentially including them in hospital orientation for new nursing staff.

Gamification in Nursing Education

Angela Malicki, MEd, MISD
Margo Preston Scott, MSN, RN-BC
Franz Henryk Vergara, PhD, DNP, RN, ONC, CCM
Marjone Zapanta Meneses, MSN, RN
Barbara Van de Castle, DNP, RN-BC, APRN-CNS, OCN
Julie Seiler, MS, RN
Madeleine Whalen, MSN/MPH, RN, CEN
Paola Goyeneche, MS
Stefanie Mann, MS, RN
The Johns Hopkins Hospital Baltimore, MD, USA

Practice Question

Clinical educators and educational course developers strive to improve learner engagement in academic and hospital settings. Adult learners in healthcare systems have unique needs, as they need to stay informed on evolving standards of practice, staff education requirements, and evidence-based practice (EBP). Traditionally, educational methods, including instructor-led with PowerPoint presentations, lectures, and didactic online modules, deliver educational content to professional nurses. These are static educational approaches that offer limited learner engagement and may compromise content retention. In our organization, course evaluations highlighted the need to leverage new technologies to optimize learners' experiences.

With the purpose of redesigning a didactic, mandatory online course for all members of our nursing staff, we explored the concept of digital gamification. We first sought to evaluate the state of the literature to answer the question:

What evidence exists on the use of interactive digital learning and gamification (I) for adult learners in healthcare education (P)?

Evidence

The project team conducted an integrative review, using search terms that included *gamification, scenario-based, digital learning*, etc., with a focus on nursing, clinical staff, resident, and other clinical personnel. The review of literature spanned across four electronic databases—PubMed, CINAHL, ERIC, and Cochrane—using the Preferred Reporting Items for Systematic Reviews and Meta-Analyses (PRISMA) and the Johns Hopkins Nursing Evidence-Based Practice (JHNEBP) model by Dang and Dearholt. The 23 studies were conducted in 10 countries between the years of 2013 and 2018. Population samples in primary reports ranged from 11 to 933 participants; however, one study from Portugal did not provide the number of participants. The literature review articles included the following evidence levels: five Level I articles, one Level II article, nine Level III articles, and eight Level V articles, all of good or high quality.

Twenty-three journal articles met the specified inclusion criteria, which included literature published between January 2013 and January 2018 and written in English with either a pre-licensure or post-licensure element that answered the practice question. The team excluded items that did not answer the practice question, did not have an online or digital gamification component, or did not have nursing involvement.

Twenty articles included content on primary reports of nursing students (n = 12), professional nurses (n = 7), and a combination of these two groups (n = 1). Of these articles, 16 supported gamification for a variety of reasons, whereas 4 studies did not show conclusive support for this approach. Eight games involved teaching content relevant to the provision of nursing clinical practice or skills, and the remaining 12 presented information on nursing theory. Thirteen articles reported on providing education in a static model, and seven studies used a dynamic approach. Ten studies reported primary results (five randomized control trials, two quality improvement projects, one quasi-experimental study, two qualitative studies), and ten described the process or reception of the game design itself.

The three remaining articles were in the form of literature reviews with nursing students (n = 2) and both nursing student and professional nurse (n = 1) populations. These reviews supported the effectiveness of gamification process, with more specific findings related to optimizing the process and offering immediate feedback. The types of immediate feedback varied; however, four immediate feedback delivery methods were recurrent: video immersion, scenario-based or virtual video, web-based games, and self-pace score testing.

Evidence synthesis resulted in overall support for the gamification process. The most support (n = 16) was in games of theory content delivered in a static manner (56%; n = 9) versus not supported (n = 4) in skill-based education following a dynamic model (50%; n = 2). Overall support for gamification was higher in theory content (69%), compared with skill content (31%). This trend was reflected in studies in which the majority of content was related to theory taught in a static manner (45%), whereas dynamic approach for skills (20%), theory (15%), and static skills (20%) were seen in the remainder of the studies.

In reviewing the evidence for this project, leveraging game design principles to optimize learner experiences was evident in most articles with good- to high-quality evidence. The learners' experiences varied based on population, educational content, and teaching methodologies.

Translation

Based on the evidence, the primary author and two of the contributing authors of this article undertook a study to measure the effects of gamification on learning outcomes when delivered to clinicians enrolled in the Clinical Technician and Clinical Nurse Extern Orientation Programs. This research was designed to gather data to measure the impact of gamification on learner engagement and retention when a clinical topic (specifically, vital signs) is delivered to the students as a board game or digital board game versus traditional lecture method with presentation slides.

The preliminary results with a small sample size indicated that 83% of learners preferred the engagement of the gamified approach over the lecture method, and those who played the game showed a 90% improvement from pre- to post-test scores. COVID-19 prevented the students from gathering to play the board game and halted the study, but it will resume once in-person classes resume.

Summary

The findings of this EBP project suggest that although the use of interactive digital learning in the form of games, gamification, and scenario-based learning has a positive effect on learner engagement and satisfaction, no study has been able to quantify any objective data on knowledge retained over time. We recommend conducting further research by testing the newest technology and interventions that may improve healthcare professionals' knowledge retention through gamification. There is also a need to develop a reliable and valid tool to objectively measure licensed healthcare professionals' knowledge retention.

An Evidence-Based Approach to Creating an EBP Culture

Stephanie Coig, MBA, BSN, RN, CPN, NEA-BC
Elena Vidrine, MSN, RN-BC, NEA-BC
Kathryn Tanet, MHA, BSN, RN, NPD-BC
Children's Hospital New Orleans, Louisiana, USA

Practice Question

Evidence-based practice (EBP) entails using the best current evidence to make clinical practice decisions. In healthcare, EBP is important because it enhances practice using the most effective care, resulting in improved outcomes. Enculturation of EBP in organizations improves patient outcomes and patient, family, and healthcare provider satisfaction. Creating an EBP culture across all disciplines is essential to reducing risk for patients, improving outcomes, achieving Magnet designation, and building a high reliability organization.

Historically within the Children's Hospital of New Orleans, practice originates from a top-to-bottom approach rather than initiation by clinical staff. However, recent changes in leadership provided the clinical staff with the opportunity to drive practice changes. In early 2019, the hospital established an interdisciplinary shared governance structure to assist the staff in leading change. The shared governance Evidence-Based Practice and Research Council completed an organizational assessment to evaluate the current resources and support for EBP. Internally, the organization lacked the structure, resources, and knowledge needed to empower staff to implement evidence-based practice changes. The Council posed the background question:

> What are the best ways to increase knowledge, confidence, and implementation of EBP (I/O) in the hospital setting (P)?

Evidence

The EBP team conducted an evidence search using PubMed and CINAHL. English-language studies of practicing nurses within the past five years met inclusion criteria. Search terms included *EBP, competency, implementation,* and *culture*. The team identified and critically appraised 11 articles using the JH-NEBP Model. Of the 11 articles, 2 were quasi-experimental, 1 mixed-method, and 8 case studies/QI projects from hospitals describing their experience with implementing EBP. Three of the studies were Level II with A/B quality, and eight were Level V with A/B quality. The evidence consistently recommended interventions such as creating a supportive EBP environment, establishing interprofessional and academic collaboration, developing an EBP education plan, building EBP into existing competencies and evaluation structure, and increasing EBP activities to promote awareness.

Much of the evidence focused on outcomes such as EBP knowledge and beliefs related to implementation of EBP, the number of completed EBP projects, and the impact of EBP projects on clinical and financial outcomes. Following the literature review but prior to the implementation of interventions, the team surveyed staff using Melnyk's EBP Beliefs and Implementation Scale. The team sent surveys to all clinical staff (1,078 people), and 859 people completed the survey. Only 56% of respondents indicated clarity about the steps of the EBP process, and 48% felt they could implement EBP sufficiently enough to change practice.

Translation

Based on the literature recommendations, the shared governance EBP and Research Council advocated with the Chief Nursing Officer and Chief Operating Officer for approval of dedicated hours for EBP work. Hospital leadership approved 12 hours per month for all clinical staff working on an EBP project. To further create a supportive EBP environment, the Council collaborated with the organization's Nurse Residency Program to assist in guiding the nurse residency EBP projects. Academic collaboration was crucial in supporting education for the Council and helping to guide the work of creating EBP structures. Three faculty members and the dean of a local nursing university are active members on the EBP and Research Council and have been valuable in mentoring members of the council. In addition, less than one year into the project, the organization partnered with the university again to secure eight hours per week of dedicated time for a Nurse Researcher.

To increase knowledge, the council developed an EBP education plan. The council received approval to contract with the Johns Hopkins Nursing Center for Evidence-Based Practice to deliver two three-day on-site workshops for the council members and nurse residency facilitators. The council created and assigned an EBP education module applicable to all clinical staff to increase awareness of the EBP process and the resources available within the organization. Lastly, the Council developed an EBP Fellowship program. The purpose of this program was to give interested clinical staff the opportunity to receive comprehensive EBP education utilizing the JHNEBP model while being mentored through their own EBP project.

The council increased EBP activities and awareness of activities through revisions to the nursing clinical ladder, marketing for the EBP Fellowship through the hospital's weekly E-news, financial support for staff attendance at conferences to disseminate EBP, and creation of an annual EBP and research day for internal dissemination of projects.

Summary

A follow-up survey was collected using Melnyk's Scale after implementation of interventions. The EBP team surveyed all clinical staff, resulting in 1,078 sent surveys and 320 completed surveys. Results indicated an improvement in the EBP Beliefs scores for 14 of the 16 statements. Specifically, 76% of respondents indicated clarity about the steps of the EBP process (up from 56%), and 66% felt they could implement EBP sufficiently enough to change practice (up from 48%).

Based on the education and promotion of the EBP Fellowship Program, 15 interdisciplinary teams entered the first cohort. In completing this evidence-based project, the team learned the importance of stakeholder buy-in from interdisciplinary department directors prior to implementation, initiating virtual learning sessions for offsite clinicians, and the importance of mentor support during EBP project implementation. The next steps for the council will be to continue program evaluation, continue offering the EBP fellowship, and disseminate this evidence-based project at the local, state, and national level.

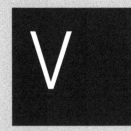

Using the JHEBP Tools

11 Lessons From Practice: Using the
   JHEBP Tools 247

Go to https://www.hopkinsmedicine.org/evidence-based-practice/ to request permission to access the forms used in *Johns Hopkins Evidence-Based Practice for Nurses and Healthcare Professionals: Model and Guidelines.*

11

Lessons From Practice: Using the JHEBP Tools

This chapter provides several examples of how teams can complete the JHEBP tools, and it gives helpful hints and guidelines to aid completion. The tools provided in this chapter reflect a brief overview of the project "EBP on Fall Prevention," by H. Farley, E. Middleton, J. Kreif, L. Nell, E. Lins, and L. Klein as an exemplar. All tools shown are copyright protected by Johns Hopkins Health System/Johns Hopkins School of Nursing.

Practice Question and Project Planning

The widely used fall prevention policy of The Johns Hopkins Hospital was due for triennial review and updates. Falls can result in serious injuries such as fractures, internal bleeding, and death. As such, falls represent a significant threat requiring current, evidence-based prevention strategies. The process of reviewing the organization's fall prevention policy included the development and management of an EBP project (Appendix A). The EBP question was: *What are best practices to prevent falls in the adult in-patient setting as evidenced by reduction in fall rates?* (Appendix B). The three-year time frame reflects the triennial review cycle of the policies.

Appendix A: PET Process Guide

The EBP team began the process with Appendix A (see Figure 11.1). It provided a starting point and a concise overview of the steps in the process.

EBP Work Plan

The PET Guide helps teams see the project timeline at a glance and can be used to track progress. The team updates it throughout the project. Where appropriate, the list pairs the steps with the coordinating appendices making it easy for teams to find the correct tools for each part of the process.

Initial EBP question: What are the best practices for adult, hospitalized patient fall prevention (including rehabilitation) in the literature from the last 3 years?

EBP team leader(s): Holley Farley

EBP team members: E. Middleton, J. Kreif, L. Nell, E. Lins, L.

Goal completion date: June 30, 2019

Complete this section after developing the EBP question using Appendix B.

Steps	Month
	Oct / Nov / Dec / Jan / Feb / Mar / Apr / May / Jun 1 / 2 / 3 / 4 / 5 / 6 / 7 / 8 / 9

Add the names of each month for added clarity

Practice Question & Project Planning
1. Recruit interprofessional team
2. Determine responsibility for project leadership
3. Schedule team meetings
4. Clarify & describe the problem (App. B)
5. Develop & refine the EBP question (App. B)
6. Determine the need for an EBP project
7. Identify stakeholders (App. C)

Determining the need for or support of an EBP project represents a critical step early in the EBP process. The "Decision tree to determine the need for an EBP project" (on the following page) guides this determination.

Evidence
8. Conduct internal & external search for

Finding meeting times for the team can be a challenge. Look for opportunities to use meetings that are already scheduled (e.g., staff or committee meetings) to minimize the need for additional meetings.

12. Develop best evidence recommendations (App. H)

Translation
13. Identify practice setting–specific recommendations (App. I)
14. Create action plan (App. I)
15. Secure support & resources to implement action plan
16. Implement action plan
17. If change is implemented, evaluate outcomes to determine if improvements have been made
18. Report results to stakeholders (App. C)
19. Identify next steps
20. Disseminate findings (App. J)

Figure 11.1 Completed Appendix A: PET Process Guide.

11 Lessons From Practice: Using the JHEBP Tools   249

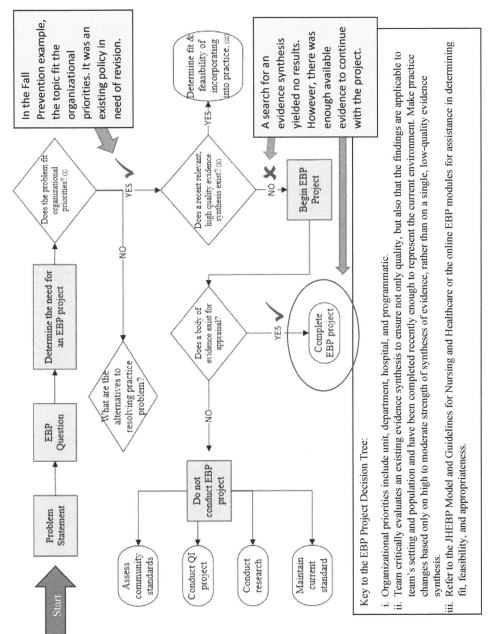

Figure 11.1 Completed Appendix A: PET Process Guide.

Appendix B: Question Development Tool

A successful EBP project depends on accurate problem identification and appropriate question selection. Teams should plan to spend substantial time completing Appendix B, and they may revisit it many times during the course of the project. Figure 11.2 shows segments of the completed Appendix B for the fall prevention policy renewal.

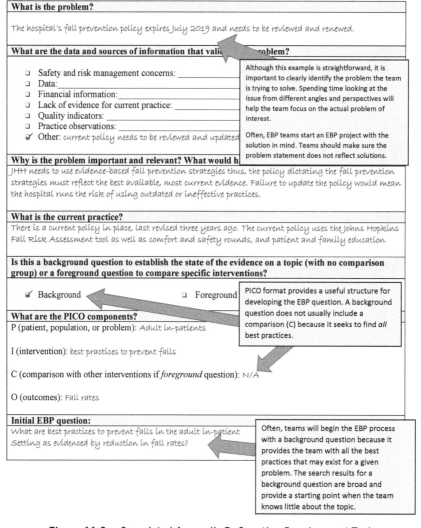

Figure 11.2   Completed Appendix B: Question Development Tool.

11 Lessons From Practice: Using the JHEBP Tools 251

List possible search terms for each part of the PICO question:	
PICO Element	Possible Search Terms
P	Inpatient, hospital, unit, ward, inpatient rehabilitation, oncolog*, neuroscience, neurointensive, acute care, acute rehabilitation
I	accidental falls, falling, falls, fall with injury
C	N/A ← *Just as is the case with the PICO, if the team has a background question they will not likely have any comparison search terms.*
O	Fall rate

What are preliminary inclusion and exclusion criteria (e.g., date, population, setting, other)?

Inclusion: English language articles published from 2015 to present	Exclusion: Non-English language articles, articles without full text availability, published before 2015, pediatric setting, outpatient setting

What evidence needs to be reviewed? (Check all that apply)

- ☑ Peer-reviewed publications (from databases such as PubMed, CINAHL, Embase)
- ☑ Standards (regulatory, professional, community)
- ☑ Clinical Practice Guidelines
- ☑ Organizational data (e.g., quality improvement or financial data, local clinical expertise, patient/family preferences)
- ☑ Evidence-based professional organization position statements
- ☑ Consensus studies (e.g., commissioned reports from the National Academy of Medicine, professional organizations, philanthropic foundations)
- ☐ Other _____

Revised EBP question: ← *As the team begins the literature review, refinement of the EBP question is common to update vocabulary or adjust specificity.*

What are measures that indicate if the EBP project is successful? (Measures may be structure, process, and/or outcome)

Falls rates- number of falls/ 1000 patient days obtained from NDNQI
Documentation compliance for fall-related items

Figure 11.2 Completed Appendix B: Question Development Tool.

Appendix C: Stakeholder Analysis and Communication Tool

Teams should spend time identifying and engaging stakeholders early in the EBP process. Failure to adequately identify and engage stakeholders could negatively impact the project. Although stakeholders may change over the life of the EBP project, the team would be well served to perform a thorough assessment before beginning. Figure 11.3 demonstrates the stakeholder analysis and communication plan (see Appendix C) for the falls project.

Stakeholder Analysis

Identify the key stakeholders:

- ☐ Manager or direct supervisor
- ☐ Finance department
- ☐ Vendors
- ☑ Patients and/or families; pa...
- ☐ Professional organizations
- ☑ Committees

- ☐ Organizational leaders
- ☑ Interdisciplinary colleagues (e.g. physicians, nutritionists, respiratory therapists, or OT/PT)
- ☐ Administrators
- ☐ Other units or departments
- ☑ Others: _frontline nurses_

The team identifies individuals who have a vested interest, role, and responsibility in the project. For example, approval of the policy falls to the clinical leaders, whereas the frontline nurses provide input and consult on content and feasibility.

Stakeholder analysis matrix: (Adapted from http://www.tools4dev.org/)

Stakeholder Name and Title:	Role: (select all that apply) Responsibility, Approval, Consult, Inform	Impact Level: (How much the project impacts them?) (minor, moderate, significant)	Influence Level: How much influence do they have over the project? (minor, moderate, significant)	What matters most to the stakeholder?	How could the stakeholder contribute to the project?	How could the stakeholder impede the project?	Strategy(s) for engaging the stakeholder:
Committees	Approval	Moderate	Significant	Safety, risk management	Approve the recommendations	Reject the recommendations	Provide evidence to support recommendations, detailed plan
Frontline nurses	Responsibility, inform, consult	Significant	Moderate	Ease of use, efficiency, safety	Pilot interventions and provide feedback	Non-adherence	Identify change champions, provide education about changes, communicate

Figure 11.3 Completed Appendix C: Stakeholder Analysis and Communication Tool.

Communication Planning

Refer to this section to guide your communications to stakeholders throughout and after completing the EBP project:

What is the purpose of the dissemination of the EBP project findings? (check all that apply)
- ☐ Raise awareness
- ☐ Promote action
- ☑ Change policy
- ☑ Change practice
- ☐ Engage stakeholders

> The reporting section will be helpful at any stage in the process but is particularly useful when the team is ready to disseminate their findings. Some sections, such as the 3 most important messages, are only evident once recommendations are determined.

What is/are the 3 most important message(s)?
1) Communication of fall risk is important and should be considered during team huddles
2) Added "consider holding a post-fall huddle"
3) Many of the current practices are considered best practices

Align key message(s) and methods with audience:

Audience	Key Messages	Method	Timing
Interdisciplinary stakeholders	The fall prevention policy will be updated to include adding consideration of risk to the team huddle and to debrief in a post-fall huddle.	email, bulletin	policy renewal July 1, 2019
Organizational Leaders	The fall prevention policy will be updated to include adding debrief in a report on fall	Staff meetings, newsletters, email, policy update bulletin	3 weeks before the policy renewal July 1, 2019
Frontline nurses	It is important to align the key message with the audience. People are interested in what the change means for them and how they may be affected. Refer back to the stakeholder matrix for what each stakeholder values. Carefully tailoring the content and message to the audience will ensure that these concerns are met.		

> Teams should consider multiple modalities for communicating the key messages. Experts recommend communicating the message six times in six different ways.

Figure 11.3 Completed Appendix C: Stakeholder Analysis and Communication Tool.

Evidence

With the assistance of the hospital Informationist, the team searched PubMed, Embase, CINAHL Plus, Cochrane Library, and JBI databases for English-language articles published from 2015 to present. Search terms were specific to the individual databases but included general terms such as *accidental falls, patient safety, falling, hospital, inpatient, prevention,* and *safety management* (Appendix B). The literature search produced 1,200 articles. After an initial title review, removing duplicate articles, and removing articles that discussed fall risk assessment tools (already in use at the organization), adult emergency department, or pediatrics, 95 articles remained. Further abstract review yielded 15 articles for appraisal. The team divided the pieces of evidence so that each article was appraised by at least two team members (Appendices E, F, and G).

Appendix E: Research Evidence Appraisal Tool

When teams are appraising research evidence (Levels I, II, III), they use Appendix E, the Research Evidence Appraisal Tool. Hint: Use Appendix D (not included in this chapter) for a quick overview for determining the level of evidence.

Figure 11.4 shows the appraisal of a Level I article using Appendix E.

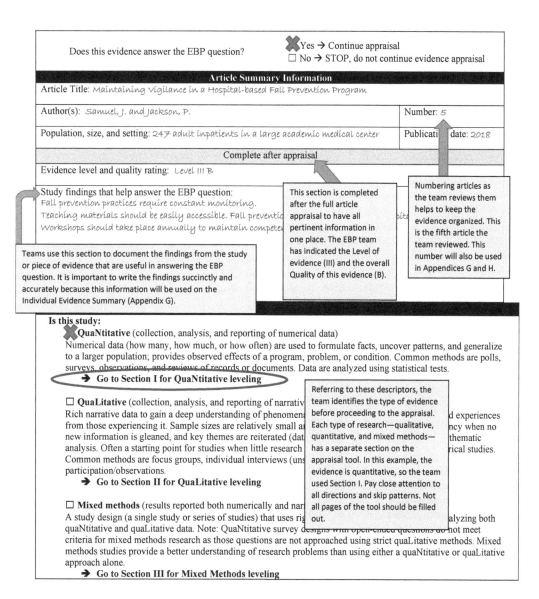

Figure 11.4 Completed Appendix E: Research Evidence Appraisal Tool.

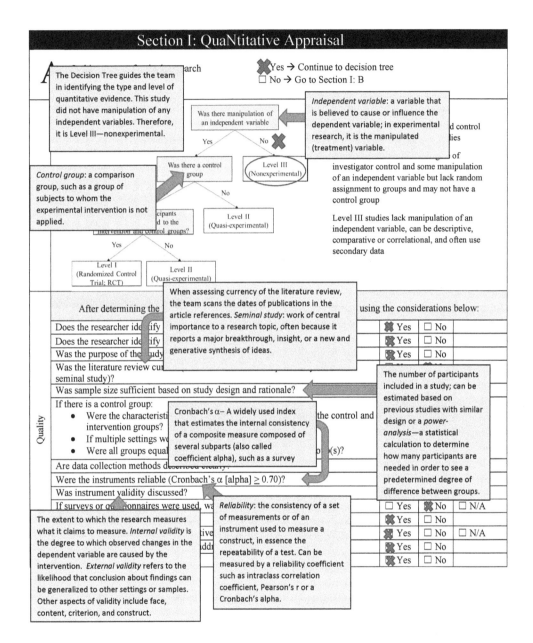

Figure 11.4 Completed Appendix E: Research Evidence Appraisal Tool.

Section I: QuaNtitative Appraisal (continued)

Circle the appropriate quality rating below:

Quality

A High quality: Consistent, generalizable results; sufficient sample size for the study design; adequate control; definitive conclusions; consistent recommendations based on comprehensive literature review that includes thorough reference to scientific evidence.

B Good quality: Reasonably consistent results; sufficient sample size for the study design; some control; fairly definitive conclusions; reasonably consistent recommendations based on fairly comprehensive literature review that includes some reference to scientific evidence.

C Low quality: Little evidence with inconsistent results; insufficient sample size for the study design; conclusions cannot be drawn.

Record findings that help answer the EBP question on page **1**

> Assessing the quality of the evidence is a subjective process based on a careful examination of the appraisal. There is no concrete number of YES answers that lead to an "A" quality rating. Rather, it involves a process of using the appraisal results together with critical thinking and discussions among team members.

Figure 11.4 Completed Appendix E: Research Evidence Appraisal Tool.

Section I: QuaNtitative Appraisal (continued)

B — Is this a summary of multiple sources of research evidence?
☐ Yes → Continue to decision tree
☐ No → Use the Nonresearch Evidence Appraisal tool (Appendix F)

Was there a comprehensive search strategy and rigorous appraisal method?
- Yes → Do the studies only include research evidence (Levels I, II or III)?
  - No → Go to the Nonresearch Evidence Appraisal Tool (Appendix F)
  - Yes → Are all studies included RCTs?
    - Yes → Level I
    - No → Do the studies include non-experimental research in addition to RCTs and/or quasi-experimental studies?
      - Yes → Level III
      - No → Level II
- No → Go to the Nonresearch Evidence Appraisal Tool (Appendix F)

Flow diagram: a visual representation of the flow of information through the different phases of a systematic review. It maps out the number of records identified, included and excluded, and the reasons for exclusions.

After determining level of evidence, determine the quality of evidence using the considerations below:

Quality	Yes	No
Were the variables of interest clearly identified?	☐ Yes	☐ No
Was the search comprehensive and reproducible? • Key terms stated • Multiple databases searched and identified • Inclusion and exclusion criteria stated	☐ Yes ☐ Yes ☐ Yes	☐ No ☐ No ☐ No
Was there a flow diagram that included the number of studies eliminated at each level of review?	☐ Yes	☐ No
Were details of included studies presented (design, sample, methods, results, outcomes, strengths, and limitations)?	☐ Yes	☐ No
Were methods for appraising the strength of evidence (level and quality) described?	☐ Yes	☐ No
Were conclusions based on results? • Results were interpreted • Conclusions flowed logically from the research question, results, and interpretation	☐ Yes ☐ Yes	☐ No ☐ No
Did the systematic review include a section addressing limitations and how they were addressed?	☐ Yes	☐ No

Figure 11.4 Completed Appendix E: Research Evidence Appraisal Tool.

	Section I: QuaNtitative Appraisal (continued)
	Circle the appropriate quality rating below:
Quality	**A High quality:** Consistent, generalizable results; sufficient sample size for the study design; adequate control; definitive conclusions; consistent recommendations based on comprehensive literature review that includes thorough reference to scientific evidence. **B Good quality:** Reasonably consistent results; sufficient sample size for the study design; some control; fairly definitive conclusions; reasonably consistent recommendations based on fairly comprehensive literature review that includes some reference to scientific evidence. **C Low quality:** Little evidence with inconsistent results; insufficient sample size for the study design; conclusions cannot be drawn.
	Record findings that help answer the EBP question on page **1**

Figure 11.4 Completed Appendix E: Research Evidence Appraisal Tool.

Section II: QuaLitative Appraisal

A	Is this a report of a single [research study]?	• This is Level III evidence Go to Section II: B

Generally, researchers establish the strength or rigor of a qualitative study through:

Credibility: confidence in the study findings demonstrated through various research strategies

Confirmability: documentation of the researchers' thinking and decisions during the study

Fittingness: whether study findings are applicable to another setting, achieved through providing rich data

After determining level [of] evidence using the considerations below:

Was there a clearly identifiable:
- Purpose?
- Research question?
- Justification for design?

Do participants have knowledge [relating to experience]?

Were characteristics of study participants [described]?

Illustrations: Researchers should provide illustrations (i.e., direct quotations of participants) from the data to show the basis of their conclusions and to ensure that participants are represented in the report.

[Was a] process used in every step of data analysis (e.g., triangulation, independent double check, member checking)? (Credibility)

[Did researchers] provide sufficient documentation of their thinking, decisions [in] the study allowing the reader to follow their decision-making [as conclusions] were formulated)? (Confirmability)

[Did researchers] provide an accurate and rich description of findings by [allowing capacity] to evaluate the analysis of data? (Fittingness)

Researchers must be self-aware of their own reactions and reflections throughout the research study. To reduce the effect of personal influence, researchers can employ several techniques such as *bracketing* (acknowledging the possible influence and intentionally setting aside conscious thoughts and decisions influenced by that mindset) and *reflexivity* (involves the researcher's self-awareness and the strategies the researcher used to manage potentially biasing factors while maintaining sensitivity to the data).

	Question	Yes	No
Quality	Does the researcher acknowledge and/or address their own role and potential influence during data collection?	☐ Yes	☐ No
	Was sampling adequate, as evidenced by achieving data saturation?		
	Does the researcher provide illustrations from the data? • If yes, do the provided illustrations support conclusions?		
	Is there congruency between the findings and the data?		
	Is there congruency between the research methodology and: • The research question(s) • Between methods to collect data • The interpretation of results	☐ Yes ☐ Yes	☐ No ☐ No
	Are discussion and conclusions congruent with the purpose and objectives, and supported by literature?	☐ Yes	☐ No
	Are conclusions drawn based on the data collected (e.g., the product of the observations or interviews)?	☐ Yes	☐ No
	Circle the appropriate quality rating below:		

Saturation: occurs when there are no new data emerging and redundancy arises-.The sufficiency of a qualitative sample is evaluated by the quality and amount of the data—not the number of participants.

Figure 11.4 Completed Appendix E: Research Evidence Appraisal Tool.

11 Lessons From Practice: Using the JHEBP Tools 261

Appendix F: Nonresearch Evidence Appraisal Tool

When teams are appraising nonresearch evidence (Levels IV, V), they use Appendix F, the Nonresearch Evidence Appraisal Tool (see Figure 11.5). Hint: Use Appendix D (not included in this chapter) for a quick overview for determining the level of evidence.

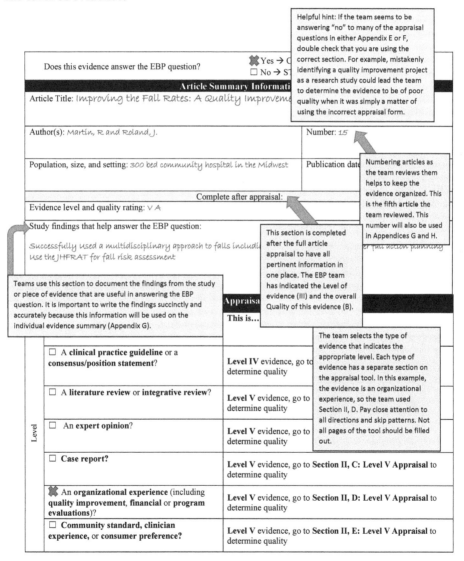

Figure 11.5 Completed Appendix F: Nonresearch Evidence Appraisal Tool.

Section I: Level IV Appraisal

Select the type of Level IV evidence

☐ **Clinical practice guidelines** (systematically developed recommendations from nationally recognized experts based on research evidence or expert consensus panel)
☐ **Consensus or position statement** (systematically developed recommendations, based on research and nationally recognized expert opinion, that guide members of a professional organization in decision-making for an issue of concern)

After selecting the type of Level IV evidence, determine the quality of evidence using the considerations below:

Are the types of evidence included identified?	☐ Yes	☐ No
Were appropriate stakeholders involved in the development of recommendations?	☐ Yes	☐ No
Are groups to which recommendations apply and do not apply clearly defined?	☐ Yes	☐ No
Does each recommendation have an identified level of evidence stated?	☐ Yes	☐ No
Are recommendations clear?	☐ Yes	☐ No

Circle the appropriate quality rating below:

A High quality: Material officially sponsored by a professional, public, or private organization or a government agency; documentation of a systematic literature search strategy; consistent results with sufficient numbers of well-designed studies; criteria-based evaluation of overall scientific strength and quality of included studies and definitive conclusions; national expertise clearly evident; developed or revised within the past five years.

B Good quality: Material officially sponsored by a professional, public, or private organization or a government agency; reasonably thorough and appropriate systematic literature search strategy; reasonably consistent results, sufficient numbers of well-designed studies; evaluation of strengths and limitations of included studies with fairly definitive conclusions; national expertise clearly evident; developed or revised within the past five years.

C Low quality: Material not sponsored by an official organization or agency; undefined, poorly defined, or limited literature search strategy; no evaluation of strengths and limitations of included studies; insufficient evidence with inconsistent results; conclusions cannot be drawn; not revised within the past five years.

Record findings that help answer the EBP question on page **1**

Figure 11.5 Completed Appendix F: Nonresearch Evidence Appraisal Tool.

11 Lessons From Practice: Using the JHEBP Tools 263

Section II: Level V Quality Appraisal

A Select the type of article:

> Literature reviews are generally descriptive and typically lack any analysis of the literature, reproducible search strategy, or rigorous evaluation method.

☐ **Literature review** (summary of selected published literature including scientific and nonscientific, such as reports of organizational experience and opinions of experts)

☐ **Integrative review** (summary of research evidence and theoretical literature; analyzes, compares themes, notes gaps in the selected literature)

> Sometimes, researchers may title or refer to integrative reviews as systematic reviews. However, closer examination reveals they combine both research evidence and theoretical literature, or nonresearch evidence.

After selecting the type of Level V evidence, determine the

Is subject matter to be reviewed clearly stated?	☐ Yes	☐ No
Is literature relevant and up-to-date (most sources are within the	☐ Yes	☐ No
Of the literature reviewed, is there a meaningful analysis of the articles included in the review?		☐ No
Are gaps in the literature identified?	☐ Yes	☐ No
Are recommendations made for future practice or study?	☐ Yes	☐ No

Circle the appropriate quality rating below:

A High quality: Expertise is clearly evident, draws definitive conclusions, and provides scientific rationale; thought leader in the field.

B Good quality: Expertise appears to be credible, draws fairly definitive conclusions, and provides logical argument for opinions.

C Low quality: Expertise is not discernable or is dubious; conclus

> Notice there are different quality guides for the various types of nonresearch evidence. Choosing an incorrect rating guide may lead the team to mislabel the quality of a piece of evidence.

Record findings that help answer the EBP

Figure 11.5   Completed Appendix F: Nonresearch Evidence Appraisal Tool.

Section II: Level V Quality Appraisal (continued)

B **Select the type of article:**

☐ **Expert opinion** (opinion of one or more individuals based on clinical expertise)

After selecting the type of Level V evidence using the considerations below:

Does the author have relevant educational background, scientific rationale;	☐ Yes	☐ No
Do they have relevant professional experience and provides logical	☐ Yes	☐ No
Have they previously published in the field?	☐ Yes	☐ No
Have they been recognized by state, regional, national or international groups for their expertise?	☐ Yes	☐ No
Are their publications well cited by others?	☐ Yes	☐ No

Expert opinion can come from one or more individuals, but does not include a consensus statement developed by a group of experts or members of a professional organization.

A web search can provide information about expertise

Circle the appropriate quality rating below:

> Teams often wonder how to differentiate between expert opinion and clinician experience. A quick internet search may tell you if the person has previously published or presented on the topic. If you are unable to find anything linking them to the topic, you may consider it clinician experience.

A High quality: Expertise is clearly evident, designated thought leader in the field.

B Good quality: Expertise appears to be credible, argument for opinions.

C Low quality: Expertise is not discernable or credible.

Record findings that help answer the EBP question on page 1

Figure 11.5 Completed Appendix F: Nonresearch Evidence Appraisal Tool.

11 Lessons From Practice: Using the JHEBP Tools   265

D Select the type of article:

☐ **Quality improvement** (cyclical method to examine workflows, processes, or systems within a specific organization)

☐ **Financial evaluation** (economic evaluation that applies analytic techniques to identify, measure, and compare the cost and outcomes of two or more alternative programs or interventions)

☐ **Program evaluation** (systematic assessment of the processes a[nd/or outcomes...] involve both quaNtitative and quaLitative methods)

After selecting the type of Level V evidence, determine the quality [below:]

Quality	
Was the aim of the project clearly stated?	
Was a formal QI method used for conducting or reporting the proje[ct (e.g.,] PDSA, SQUIRE 2.0)?	
Was the method fully described?	
Were process or outcome measures identified?	
Were results fully described?	
Was interpretation clear and appropriate?	
Are components of cost/benefit or cost effectiveness data describe[d?]	N/A

Circle the appropriate quality ra[ting:]

A High quality: Clear aims and objectives; consistent results acros[s multiple settings;] improvement or financial evaluation methods used; definitive conc[lusions;] thorough reference to scientific evidence.

B Good quality: Clear aims and objectives; formal quality improv[ement;] consistent results in a single setting; reasonably consistent recomm[endations based on fairly comprehensive] evidence.

C Low quality: Unclear or missing aims and objectives; inconsistent results; poorly defined quality improvement/financial analysis method; recommendations cannot be made.

Record findings that help answer the EBP question on page **1**

One of the biggest challenges teams may face when appraising evidence is determining if something is research or quality improvement. Keep in mind, QI:

✓ Seeks to improve a program, system, or process.
✓ Does not increase risk to patients (aside from privacy or confidentiality) and does not require consent
✓ Uses an adaptive, iterative project design
✓ Is designed to implement knowledge or assess an established process or program without the option to opt in or out

When in doubt, look to the author's purpose statement for clarity. Was the intent to improve something in their organization (QI) or to generate new knowledge for broad application (research)?

Figure 11.5 Completed Appendix F: Nonresearch Evidence Appraisal Tool.

Appendix G: Individual Evidence Summary Form

As the EBP team completes the appraisal of evidence, each article or piece of evidence should be entered into Appendix G. This becomes the team's reference and synopsis of the evidence reviewed. Remember that each piece of evidence should be appraised by more than one member of the team, and together they reach a consensus on level and quality. Some groups may decide to enter each article as it is read and discussed, whereas others may wait until all articles have been appraised. Either way is acceptable. Figure 11.6 provides a snapshot of Appendix G and shows only three of the articles reviewed. Note that evidence rated C-quality should not be used or transferred to Appendix G. The team should not rely on low-quality evidence to make decisions.

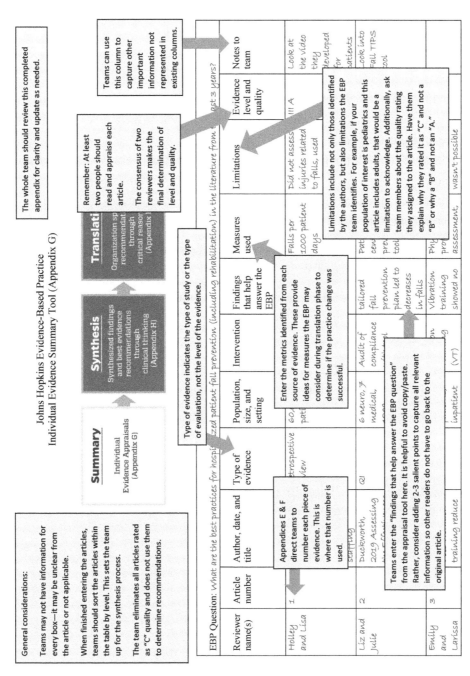

Figure 11.6 Completed Appendix G: Individual Evidence Summary Tool.

Appendix H: Synthesis and Recommendations Tool

Once Appendix G is completed, the team moves into evidence synthesis. The synthesis process is described in Appendix H. Using this tool, the team outlines the overall quality of the evidence to answer the EBP question, including the number of sources for each level. This appendix is also where the team, through reasoning, evaluates evidence for consistency across findings; evaluates the meaning and relevance of the findings; and merges findings that may either enhance the team's knowledge or generate new insights, perspectives, and understandings. In Appendix H the team identifies the best evidence recommendations. See Figure 11.7 for a completed Appendix H.

During the synthesis process, the team developed the following best evidence recommendations (Appendix H):

- Tailoring patient education to their individual fall risks is found to increase patient awareness of fall risk.
- Individualized patient and family education is an important strategy for fall prevention.
- There is limited information regarding the use of video monitoring.
- A multidisciplinary approach strengthens fall prevention efforts.
- Team huddles and debriefs increase knowledge and improve communication around fall prevention.
- Further research is needed on the use of bed alarms for fall prevention.

11 Lessons From Practice: Using the JHEBP Tools   269

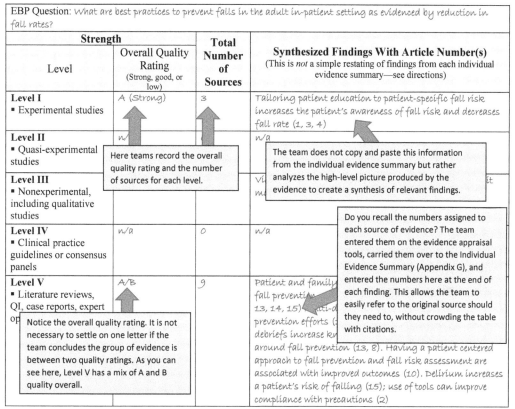

Figure 11.7   Completed Appendix H: Synthesis and Recommendations Tool.

Where does the evidence show consistency?
- Individualized patient education plan.
- Multi-disciplinary approach to fall prevention.
- An appropriate risk assessment is associated with better outcomes for falls.
- Delirium increases a patient's risk of falling.

Where does the evidence show inconsistency?
There is good but conflicting evidence for remote video monitoring for fall prevention and the use of bed alarms for fall prevention.

Best evidence recommendations (taking into consideration quantity, consistency, and strength of the evidence):
Policies should tailor patient education with an individualized approach.
Multi-disciplinary inclusion in fall prevention.
Use fall risk assessment tools.
Monitor for cognition changes and delirium.
More research is needed for video monitoring and bed alarms.

Based on your synthesis, select the statement that best describes the overall characteristics of the body of evidence?
☐ **Strong & compelling evidence, consistent results→** Recommendations are reliable; evaluate for organizational translation.
☑ **Good & consistent results→** Recommendations may be reliable; evaluate for risk and organizational translation.
☐ **Good but conflicting results→** Unable to establish best practice based on current evidence; evaluate risk, consider further investigation for new evidence, develop a research study, or discontinue the project.
☐ **Little or no evidence→** Unable to establish best practice based on current evidence; consider further investigation for new evidence, develop a research study, or discontinue the project.

Figure 11.7 Completed Appendix H: Synthesis and Recommendations Tool.

Translation

The EBP team recommended, and the appropriate oversight committees approved, changes to the policy. The revised policy reflects an individualized approach to patient education regarding fall prevention. Additions to the policy included: communication of fall risk "during team huddle," "initiate remote video monitoring (if available)," and "consider holding a post-fall huddle." The EBP project also confirmed that many of the current practices in policy reflect evidence-based, best practices in the literature. The policy will continue to include cognition in the fall risk assessment and consider further investigation of delirium screening as appropriate. The EBP team recommended no practice change on use of bed alarms for fall prevention. Further research on use of exit alarms for fall prevention is necessary. The fall prevention community will also continue to monitor the literature surrounding post-fall debriefing and remote video monitoring for fall prevention. The policy change was facilitated through the appropriate channels, and education on these changes was provided to nurses, physicians, and other providers.

The EBP team will continue to monitor policy and practice implications on nurse-sensitive patient outcomes of falls and falls with injury.

Appendix I: Action Planning Tool

Translating EBP findings into practice is multifaceted and is the fundamental part of the PET process—the reason EBP projects are undertaken. Once the team has identified organization-specific recommendations, the next step is to plan for implementation. Appendix I provides an opportunity to identify strengths in the internal environment, potential barriers, and plans for mitigation. In addition, it prompts the team to confirm the available resources and funding prior to rollout. Finally, Appendix I guides the team to identify outcome measures and group the action planning tasks into high-level deliverables. Figure 11.8 shows the completed Appendix I based on the exemplar.

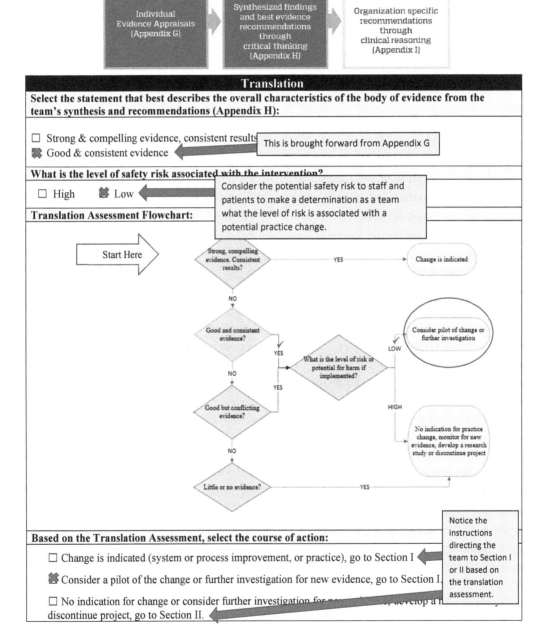

Figure 11.8 Completed Appendix I: Action Planning Tool.

Section I: If change is indicated, generate organization-specific recommendations by assessing the best-evidence recommendations for feasibility, fit, and acceptability:	
Feasibility Extent to which the team evaluates and believes that the change is low risk, doable, and can be successfully implemented within a given organization or setting.	☒ The chang... ☒ Few, if an... effort. and res... ☒ Sponsors... endorse and s... *The team used this list to assess evidence-based recommendations and checks each box when the concept has been addressed to ensure the fit, feasibility and acceptability of their organization-specific recommendations.*
Fit Compatibility of a change with end user workflow and consumer expectations; and/or the perceived relevance of the change in addressing the problem and in answering the PICO question within a given practice setting.	☒ The change aligns with unit and/or departmental priorities. ☒ The change is suitable and seems like a good match with end-user workflow. ☒ The change is applicable to the problem and answers the PICO question.
Acceptability Extent to which stakeholders and organizational leadership perceive the change to be agreeable, palatable, satisfactory and reasonable.	☒ The change aligns with organizational priorities. ☒ The change meets the approval of stakeholders and organizational leadership. ☒ Stakeholders and leaders like and welcome the change and find it appealing.
Organization-specific recommendations:	
We recommend continuing to assess cognition in the fall risk assessment and consider further investigation of delirium screening as an institution. *We recommend the policy reflect patient education with an individual specific interventions to increase patient involvement.* *We recommend further investigation into the use of video monitoring* *We recommend continued use of the JHFRAT.* *We recommend maintaining the policy with a few minor adjust...*	*After determining they had good and consistent evidence and determining the fit, feasibility, and acceptability of the best evidence recommendations, the team developed organization-specific recommendations and listed them here. These recommendations flow directly from the best evidence recommendations on Appendix H.*
Section II: When a change or pilot is not indicated, what, if any, next steps does the EBP team recommend?	
N/A	

Figure 11.8 Completed Appendix I: Action Planning Tool.

Action Planning

Complete the following activities to ensure successful implementation:

- ✖ Secure a project leader
- ✖ Identify change champions
- ✖ Consider whether translation activities require different or additional members
- ✖ Identify objectives and related tasks
- ✖ Determine dates to complete tasks
- ✖ Identify observable pre and post measures

> Often, translation requires different team members than those who worked on the EBP project. It is not uncommon for members to be added at this stage.

Identify strengths that can be leveraged to overcome barriers to ensure the success of the change:

Resources or Strengths	Barriers	Plan to Overcome Barriers by Leveraging Strengths as Appropriate
Existing policy	Committee by-in or approval of changes	Bring a representative of key committees in on the project and let them see the evidence collected
Strong core group of nurse educators	Too busy with orientation to handle training staff on changes	Begin education a few weeks prior to July 1.
Existing newsletter for dissemination	Not everyone reads the newsletter	Disseminate changes in a variety of modalities to capture all readers

> Identifying potential resources and barriers prior to implementation allows the team to take a positive approach and take time to develop plans to overcome those barriers. It is helpful to match a resource or strength with every barrier (of course, you can have more than one strength for each barrier, too).

Which of the following will be affected by this change? (*Select all that apply*)

☐ Electronic health record ☐ Workflow ☒ Policies and/or procedures ☐ Other _____

Identify and secure the resources and/or funding required for translation and implementation: (*Check all that apply*)

- ☐ Personnel costs
- ☐ Supplies/equipment
- ☐ Technology
- ☐ Education or further training
- ☐ Content or external experts
- ☐ Dissemination costs (conference costs, travel)
- ☐ Other: _____

Figure 11.8 Completed Appendix I: Action Planning Tool.

Outcome Measurement Plan					
What is/are the goal(s) of the project?	To ensure the fall prevention policy is up-to-date and reflects the best available evidence to prevent falls		**Desired completion date:**	June 31, 2019	
How will you know if you are successful?	**Types of Outcomes**	**Selected Metrics**		**Source**	**Frequency**
	☒ **Clinical** (e.g., vital signs, infection rates, fall rates, adverse events)	Falls/100 patient days		EMR	Quarterly
	☐ **Functional** (e.g., activities of daily living, quality of life, self-medication administration)	The outcome measurement plan was developed using the foreground question and PICO from Appendix B. Teams can select more than one outcome to track but should keep the number low to make the measurement process manageable.			
	☐ **Perceptual** (e.g., satisfaction, care experience, timeliness of response)				
	☐ **Process/Intervention** (e.g., care coordination, immunization, bereavement support)				
	☐ **Organization/Unit-Based** (e.g., staffing levels, length of stay, readmissions)				
Work Breakdown Structure					
High Level Deliverable	**Associated Tasks and Sub-Tasks**		**Start Date**	**End Date**	**Responsible Party**
Revised Policy	• Identify person to update policy • Convene stakeholders to review changes • Disseminate policy changes to hospital		May 1, 2019	June 31, 2019	Falls committee

Figure 11.8 Completed Appendix I: Action Planning Tool.

Appendix J: Publication Guide

The final step in any EBP project is dissemination. It is important to communicate practice changes and results of EBP projects both internally and externally. Recall that the Stakeholder Analysis and Communication Tool (Appendix C) guides the team in crafting and delivering key messages. Teams should consult Appendix C for internal dissemination. Though not a part of this chapter, The Publication Guide (Appendix J) targets an external audience and assists groups in publishing the EBP project and findings.

The tools provided in the JHNEBP Model provide structure and guidance to teams completing evidence-based practice projects. The tools are intended to walk the team through each step of the process and are meant to be completed in sequence. However, teams may sometimes need to step back and return to previously completed appendices. For example, after an intial review of the evidence, the team may decide to change the EBP question from background to foreground, requiring a return to Appendix B. Additionally, teams will return to Appendix C to craft messages for dissemination.

VI

Appendices

A PET Process Guide 279

B Question Development Tool 283

C Stakeholder Analysis and Communication Tool . . . 289

D Hierarchy of Evidence Guide 295

E Research Evidence Appraisal Tool 297

F Nonresearch Evidence Appraisal Tool 307

G Individual Evidence Summary Tool 315

H Synthesis and Recommendations Tool 319

I Translation and Action Planning Tool 325

J Publication Guide 333

Go to https://www.hopkinsmedicine.org/evidence-based-practice/ to request permission to access the forms used in *Johns Hopkins Evidence-Based Practice for Nurses and Healthcare Professionals: Model and Guidelines*.

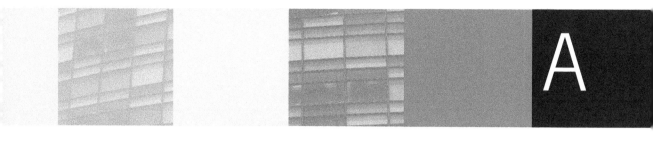

PET Process Guide

Practice Question → Evidence → Translation

Appendix A: PET Process Guide

EBP Work Plan

Initial EBP question:

EBP team leader(s):
EBP team members:
Goal completion date:

Steps	Month
	1	2	3	4	5	6	7	8	9

Practice Question & Project Planning
1. Recruit interprofessional team
2. Determine responsibility for project leadership
3. Schedule team meetings
4. Clarify & describe the problem (App. B)
5. Develop & refine the EBP question (App. B)
6. Determine the need for an EBP project
7. Identify stakeholders (App. C)

Evidence
8. Conduct internal & external search for evidence
9. Appraise the level & quality of each piece of evidence (Apps. E/F)
10. Summarize the individual evidence (App. G)
11. Synthesize findings (App. H)
12. Develop best evidence recommendations (App. H)

Translation
13. Identify practice setting–specific recommendations (App. I)
14. Create action plan (App. I)
15. Secure support & resources to implement action plan
16. Implement action plan
17. If change is implemented, evaluate outcomes to determine if improvements have been made
18. Report results to stakeholders (App. C)
19. Identify next steps
20. Disseminate findings (App. J)

©2022 Johns Hopkins Health System/Johns Hopkins School of Nursing

Appendix A: PET Process Guide   281

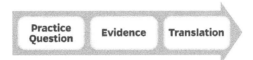

Decision tree to determine the need for an EBP project

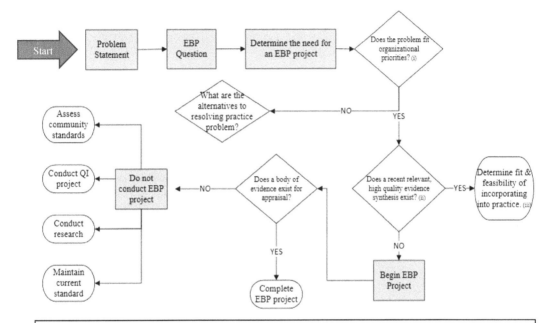

Key to the EBP Project Decision Tree:

i. Organizational priorities include unit, department, hospital, and programmatic.
ii. Team critically evaluates an existing evidence synthesis to ensure not only quality, but also that the findings are applicable to team's setting and population and have been completed recently enough to represent the current environment. Make practice changes based only on high to moderate strength of syntheses of evidence, rather than on a single, low-quality evidence synthesis.
iii. Refer to the JHEBP Model and Guidelines for Nursing and Healthcare or the online EBP modules for assistance in determining fit, feasibility, and appropriateness.

©2022 Johns Hopkins Health System/Johns Hopkins School of Nursing

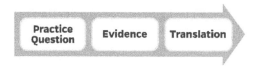

Directions for Use of the PET Process Guide

Purpose: The PET Process Guide is a tool to plan each step of the EBP process using the related Appendix, as indicated.

See Chapter 11, Lessons from Practice, for examples of completed tools.

EBP Project Plan: The project plan is dynamic, and the team should revisit due dates for each step throughout the EBP project. Best practice is to start with the desired completion date and work backward to determine a due date for each step. Shade the month box(es) that correspond to the completion date for each step in a row. Shaded boxes across rows may overlap. The team can convert the numbered months to month name. Where applicable, the corresponding EBP Appendix tool is noted.

Decision tree to determine the need for an EBP project:

The EBP decision tree guides the team in determining if an EBP project is the appropriate inquiry approach and is value-added. *Note:* Evidence must exist to conduct an *evidence*-based practice project. If an evidence-based practice synthesis of evidence exists (internally or externally to the organization) and the team determines it is high-quality, recent, and applicable to the situation or population, the team moves to recommendations and translation.

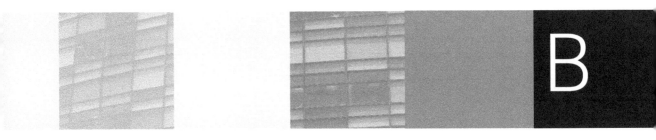

Question Development Tool

Appendix B: Question Development Tool

What is the problem?

What are the data and sources of information that validate the problem?

- ☐ Safety and risk management concerns: _____
- ☐ Data: _____
- ☐ Financial information: _____
- ☐ Lack of evidence for current practice: _____
- ☐ Quality indicators: _____
- ☐ Practice observations: _____
- ☐ Other: _____

Why is the problem important and relevant? What would happen if it were not addressed?

What is the current practice?

Is this a background question to establish the state of the evidence on a topic (with no comparison group) or a foreground question to compare specific interventions?

☐ Background   ☐ Foreground

What are the PICO components?

P (patient, population, or problem):

I (intervention):

C (comparison with other interventions if *foreground* question):

O (outcomes):

Initial EBP question:

List possible search terms for each part of the PICO question:

©2022 Johns Hopkins Health System/Johns Hopkins School of Nursing

Appendix B: Question Development Tool

PICO Element	Possible Search Terms
P	
I	
C	
O	

What are preliminary inclusion and exclusion criteria (e.g., date, population, setting, other)?

Inclusion:	Exclusion:

What evidence needs to be reviewed? (Check all that apply)

☐ Peer-reviewed publications (from databases such as PubMed, CINAHL, Embase)
☐ Standards (regulatory, professional, community)
☐ Clinical Practice Guidelines
☐ Organizational data (e.g., quality improvement or financial data, local clinical expertise, patient/family preferences)
☐ Evidence-based professional organization position statements
☐ Consensus studies (e.g., commissioned reports from the National Academy of Medicine, professional organizations, philanthropic foundations)
☐ Other _____

Revised EBP question:

What are measures that indicate if the EBP project is successful? (Measures may be structure, process, and/or outcome)

©2022 Johns Hopkins Health System/Johns Hopkins School of Nursing

Directions for Use of the Question Development Tool

Purpose: This form guides the EBP team to develop an answerable EBP question. It is meant to be fluid and dynamic as the team engages in the PICO question development process. As the team becomes familiar with the evidence base for the topic of interest, they revisit, revise, and/or refine the question, search terms, search strategy, and sources of evidence.

> See Chapter 11, Lessons from Practice, for examples of completed tools.

What is the problem?

Describe and specify the problem that needs to be addressed. What led the team to question this practice? Validate the problem statement with staff who experience it day to day. It is important for the interprofessional team to work through the problem definition process together to probe the problem description, reflect, gather information, observe current practice, and listen to clinicians' perspectives. This team deliberation ensures the problem statement defines the actual problem rather than a solution and guides the type of measure(s) they will use to determine if the intervention results in improvements once implemented.

What are the data and sources of information that validate the problem?

Confirm the problem with concrete, rather than anecdotal, information. Concrete information exists in the form of staff or patient safety concerns, data demonstrating unsatisfactory process or outcome measures, financial reports, identification of the lack of evidence for a current practice, or unsatisfactory quality indicators. Formal information or observations may demonstrate variations within the practice setting or variation within the community. These elements are not mutually exclusive, and the problem may be evidenced in multiple areas.

Why is the problem important and relevant? What would happen if it were not addressed?

Establishing a sense of importance and urgency for a practice problem can help build support for the EBP project and on-board other stakeholders. Emphasize why the problem must be addressed and the potential consequences of not doing so. This is the place to establish your "burning platform" for practice change.

What is the current practice?

Define the current practice as it relates to the problem by identifying the gap or performance issue. Think about current policies and procedures as well as adherence to these guidelines. What is commonly considered acceptable among the staff related to their daily practice? Do policy and practice align? What do you see?

Is this a background question to establish the evidence on a topic (with no comparison group) or a foreground question to compare specific interventions?

Select if you are intending to write a background or foreground question. Background questions are broad and produce a wide range of evidence to establish best practices when the team has little knowledge, experience, or expertise in the area of interest. Background questions do not include a "comparison" group. Foreground questions are focused, with specific comparison of two or more ideas or interventions. Foreground questions often flow from an initial background question and evidence review.

What are the PICO components?

Complete each section. Definitions of each PICO element are included below.

P (patient, population, problem): This may include characteristics such as age, sex, setting, ethnicity, condition, disease, type of patient or community.

I (intervention): This can be a best practice statement or include a specific treatment, medication, education, diagnostic test, or care practice.

C (comparison): Not applicable for background questions. For foreground questions, comparisons are typically with current practice or an intervention identified in the evidence.

O (outcomes): structure, process, or outcomes measures that indicate the success of evidence translation. More than one measure can be listed; examples include structure (e.g., adequacy of resources, space, people, training), process (e.g., care coordination, adherence to protocols for care, performance), or outcomes (e.g., satisfaction scores or retention, fall rates, rates of disease in a population).

Initial EBP Question:

Combine each element of the PICO to create an answerable EBP question. The initial question is refined throughout the PET process.

List possible search terms for each part of the PICO question:

Select concepts from each PICO component to identify search terms. Mapping search terms to each component aids the evidence search; ensure terms are neither too broad nor too narrow. Brainstorm common synonyms for each concept. Be sure to consider alternate spellings or terms used in different countries (e.g., "ward" vs. "unit") as well as brand names of specific interventions. It may be appropriate to leave some of the rows blank (e.g., the O in PICO) in order to avoid building solutions into the search itself (e.g., words like "reduction" will only provide evidence that exhibited reductions in the outcome of interest and may miss evidence with no change or even an increase).

What are preliminary inclusion and exclusion criteria (e.g., publication date, population, and setting)?

As a team, list initial characteristics you want to include or exclude from your evidence search (for example you may want to include student nurses but do not want to include post-licensure nurses). This will help to ensure the team has a mutual understanding of the scope of the project. The group should revisit the list throughout the process to provide further clarifications and refine evidence search results.

What evidence needs to be reviewed?

Select the types of evidence you intend to gather based on the PICO and initial EBP question. This will guide you to the appropriate sources to begin the search.

Revised EBP question:

Often the question that you start with will not be the final EBP question. Needed revisions to the EBP question may not be evident until after the initial evidence review; examples include revision to the background question or a change from a background to a foreground question. Additionally, preliminary reviews of the evidence may indicate a need to focus or broaden the question, update terminology, and/or consider additional measures of success.

What are measures that indicate if the EBP project is successful? (Measures may be structure, process and/or outcome)

It is essential to consider a measurement plan from the onset of an EBP project. As a team, reflect on how you will determine project success. Success can be captured in many ways, and measures can include:

- Structure measures that describe the physical or organizational environment (e.g., nurse-patio ratios)
- Outcome measures that occur at the conclusion of a project (e.g., number of safety events)
- Process measures that are gathered throughout to track progress toward the goals (e.g., use of a new tool or protocol)

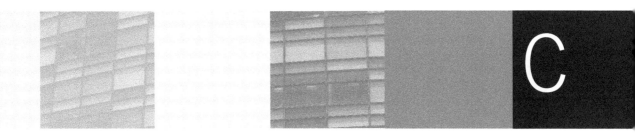

Stakeholder Analysis and Communication Tool

Appendix C: Stakeholder Analysis and Communication Tool

Stakeholder Analysis

Identify the key stakeholders:

- ☐ Manager or direct supervisor
- ☐ Finance department
- ☐ Vendors
- ☐ Patients and/or families; patient and family advisory committee
- ☐ Professional organizations
- ☐ Committees

- ☐ Organizational leaders
- ☐ Interdisciplinary colleagues (e.g., physicians, nutritionists, respiratory therapists, or OT/PT)
- ☐ Administrators
- ☐ Other units or departments
- ☐ Others: _____

Stakeholder analysis matrix:

Stakeholder Name and Title:	Role: (select all that apply) Responsibility, Approval, Consult, Inform	Impact Level: How much does the project impact them? (minor, moderate, significant)	Influence Level: How much influence do they have over the project? (minor, moderate, significant)	What matters most to the stakeholder?	How could the stakeholder contribute to the project?	How could the stakeholder impede the project?	Strategy(s) for engaging the stakeholder:

(Adapted from http://www.tools4dev.org/)

©2022 Johns Hopkins Health System/Johns Hopkins School of Nursing

Appendix C: Stakeholder Analysis and Communication Tool

Communication Planning

Refer to this section to guide your communications to stakeholders throughout and after completing the EBP project.

What is the purpose of the dissemination of the EBP project findings? (check all that apply)

- ☐ Raise awareness
- ☐ Promote action
- ☐ Change policy
- ☐ Change practice
- ☐ Engage stakeholders
- ☐ Inform stakeholders
- ☐ Other: _____

What are the three most important messages?

Align key message(s) and methods with audience:

Audience	Key Messages	Method	Timing
Interdisciplinary stakeholders			
Organizational leadership			
Frontline nurses			
Departmental leadership			
External community			
Other			

©2022 Johns Hopkins Health System/Johns Hopkins School of Nursing

Directions for Use of the Stakeholder Analysis and Communication Tool

> See Chapter 11, Lessons from Practice, for examples of completed tools.

Purpose:

The EBP team uses this form to identify key stakeholders. Key stakeholders are persons, groups, or departments that have an interest in, concern about, or stake in your project. This may include approval, subject matter expertise, or resources. Communicate with stakeholders early in the process and keep them updated on progress to ensure their buy-in for implementation.

Because stakeholders may change at different steps of the process, we recommend that you review this form as you proceed from step to step in your action plan.

The communication planning section is useful to promote communication throughout the EBP project process. Ideally, complete the communication section toward the end of the EBP project when the team has identified organization-specific recommendations.

Identify the key stakeholders (broad categories):

Consider the various areas, departments, groups, or organizations that may be impacted by or have influence over the proposed practice change.

Stakeholder analysis matrix:

Using the prompts from above, identify the five to seven stakeholders who can most affect (or who will be most affected by) the results and who can influence the success of the translation work. Consider which of the four roles each stakeholder may play in your action planning and translation work. The possible **roles** are:

- Responsibility – Completes identified tasks. Recommending authority
- Approval – Signs off on recommendations. May veto
- Consult – Provides input (e.g., subject matter experts). No decision-making authority
- Inform – Notified of progress and changes. No input on decisions

Remember that one stakeholder may fill different roles, depending on the action. Completion of the Stakeholder Analysis Tool will help clarify roles and responsibilities. The descriptions of responsibilities for each role provided on the form will be helpful in this process.

EBP teams should consider the amount of **impact** the project may have on the stakeholder and the amount of **influence** the stakeholder can have on the project's success. Identifying the ways the stakeholder can both **contribute** to and **impede** the project's success as well as how best to **engage** the stakeholder allows teams to develop plans to optimize the best outcomes.

Align key message(s) and methods with audience:

Audience: Think about the project recommendations. Identify the end users—who is your audience? Revisit the Stakeholder Analysis Tool to confirm stakeholders and key messages they need to receive. What do you want the target audience(s) to hear, know, and understand?

Key Messages: Messages should be clear, succinct, personalized to the audience, benefit-focused, actionable, and repeated 3-6 different times and ways.

Method: Communication can occur on many levels using varying strategies.
- Internal dissemination methods can include newsletters, internal website, private social media groups, journal clubs, grand rounds, staff meetings, tool kits, podcasts and lunch-and-learns.
- External dissemination can be in the form of conference poster and podium presentations, peer-reviewed articles, opinion pieces, letters to the editor, book chapters, interviews, or social media (blogs, Twitter, YouTube).

Timing: When will your message have the most impact? Consider the audience and time communication when the content may be most relevant to them and their priorities. Also, keep in mind events such as holidays and the academic calendar that can distract audiences' attention.

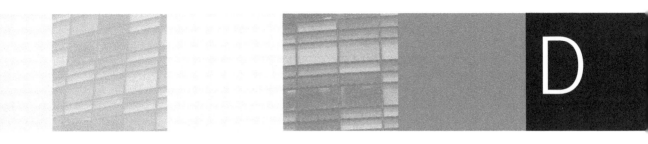

Hierarchy of Evidence Guide

Note: Refer to the appropriate Evidence Appraisal Tool (Research [Appendix E] or Nonresearch [Appendix F]) to determine quality ratings.

Appendix D: Hierarchy of Evidence Guide

Evidence Level	Types of Evidence
Level I (Research Evidence — Appendix E)	• Experimental study, randomized controlled trial (RCT) • Explanatory mixed methods design that includes only a Level I quaNtitative study • Systematic review of RCTs, with or without meta-analysis
Level II (Research Evidence — Appendix E)	• Quasi-experimental study • Explanatory mixed methods design that includes only a Level II quaNtitative study • Systematic review of a combination of RCTs and quasi-experimental studies, or quasi-experimental studies only, with or without meta-analysis
Level III (Research Evidence — Appendix E)	• Nonexperimental study • Systematic review of a combination of RCTs, quasi-experimental and nonexperimental studies, or nonexperimental studies only, with or without meta-analysis. • Exploratory, convergent, or multiphasic mixed methods studies • Explanatory mixed methods design that includes only a Level III quaNtitative study • QuaLitative study • Systematic review of quaLitative studies with or without meta-synthesis
Level IV (Nonresearch Evidence — Appendix F)	Opinion of respected authorities and/or nationally recognized expert committees or consensus panels based on scientific evidence. Includes: • Clinical practice guidelines • Consensus panels/position statements
Level V (Nonresearch Evidence — Appendix F)	Based on experiential and non-research evidence. Includes: • Scoping reviews • Integrative reviews • Literature reviews • Quality improvement, program or financial evaluation • Case reports • Opinion of nationally recognized expert(s) based on experiential evidence

©2022 Johns Hopkins Health System/Johns Hopkins School of Nursing

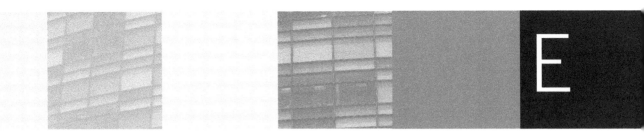

Research Evidence Appraisal Tool

Does this evidence answer the EBP question?	☐ Yes → Continue appraisal
	☐ No → STOP, do not continue evidence appraisal

Article Summary Information

Article Title:	
Author(s):	Number:
Population, size, and setting:	Publication date:

Complete after appraisal

Evidence level and quality rating:

Study findings that help answer the EBP question:

Article Appraisal Workflow

Is this study:

☐ **QuaNtitative** (collection, analysis, and reporting of numerical data)
Numerical data (how many, how much, or how often) are used to formulate facts, uncover patterns, and generalize to a larger population; provides observed effects of a program, problem, or condition. Common methods are polls, surveys, observations, and reviews of records or documents. Data are analyzed using statistical tests.
→ For **QuaNtitative** leveling of a **single** research study, go to Section IA
→ For **QuaNtitative** leveling of **multiple** research studies, go to Section IIB

☐ **QuaLitative** (collection, analysis, and reporting of narrative data)
Rich narrative data to gain a deep understanding of phenomena, meanings, perceptions, concepts, and experiences from those experiencing it. Sample sizes are relatively small and determined by the point of redundancy when no new information is gleaned, and key themes are reiterated (data saturation). Data are analyzed using thematic analysis. Often a starting point for studies when little research exists; may use results to design empirical studies. Common methods are focus groups, individual interviews (unstructured or semi-structured), and participation/observations.
→ For **QuaLitative** leveling of a **single** research study, go to Section IIA
→ For **QuaLitative** leveling of **multiple** research studies, go to Section IIB

☐ **Mixed methods** (results reported both numerically and narratively)
A study design (a single study or series of studies) that uses rigorous procedures in collecting and analyzing both quaNtitative and quaLitative data. *Note*: QuaNtitative survey designs with open-ended questions do not meet criteria for mixed methods research because those questions are not approached using strict quaLitative methods. Mixed methods studies provide a better understanding of research problems than using either a quaNtitative or quaLitative approach alone.
→ For **Mixed Methods** leveling of **single** and **mixed** studies review go to Section III

Section I: QuaNtitative Appraisal

A Is this a report of a single research study?
☐ Yes → Continue to decision tree
☐ No → Go to Section I: B

Level

```
                    Was there manipulation of
                     an independent variable
                    /                        \
                  Yes                         No
                   |                          |
            Was there a control           Level III
                  group                 (Nonexperimental)
              /         \
            Yes          No
             |            |
    Were study participants     Level II
    randomly assigned to the  (Quasi-experimental)
  intervention and control groups?
         /        \
       Yes         No
        |           |
     Level I     Level II
  (Randomized Control  (Quasi-experimental)
    Trial; RCT)
```

Level I studies include randomized control trials (RCTs) or experimental studies

Level II studies have some degree of investigator control and some manipulation of an independent variable but lack random assignment to groups and may not have a control group

Level III studies lack manipulation of an independent variable; can be descriptive, comparative, or correlational; and often use secondary data

Quality

After determining the level of evidence, determine the quality of evidence using the considerations below:

Does the researcher identify what is known and not known about the problem?	☐ Yes	☐ No	
Does the researcher identify how the study will address any gaps in knowledge?	☐ Yes	☐ No	
Was the purpose of the study clearly presented?	☐ Yes	☐ No	
Was the literature review current (most sources within the past five years or a seminal study)?	☐ Yes	☐ No	
Was sample size sufficient based on study design and rationale?	☐ Yes	☐ No	
If there is a control group: • Were the characteristics and/or demographics similar in both the control and intervention groups?	☐ Yes	☐ No	☐ N/A
• If multiple settings were used, were the settings similar?	☐ Yes	☐ No	☐ N/A
• Were all groups equally treated except for the intervention group(s)?	☐ Yes	☐ No	☐ N/A
Are data collection methods described clearly?	☐ Yes	☐ No	
Were the instruments reliable (Cronbach's α [alpha] ≥ 0.70)?	☐ Yes	☐ No	☐ N/A
Was instrument validity discussed?	☐ Yes	☐ No	☐ N/A
If surveys or questionnaires were used, was the response rate ≥ 25%?	☐ Yes	☐ No	☐ N/A
Were the results presented clearly?	☐ Yes	☐ No	
If tables were presented, was the narrative consistent with the table content?	☐ Yes	☐ No	☐ N/A
Were study limitations identified and addressed?	☐ Yes	☐ No	
Were conclusions based on results?	☐ Yes	☐ No	

©2022 Johns Hopkins Health System/Johns Hopkins School of Nursing

	Section I: QuaNtitative Appraisal (continued)
	Circle the appropriate quality rating below:
Quality	**A High quality:** Consistent, generalizable results; sufficient sample size for the study design; adequate control; definitive conclusions; consistent recommendations based on comprehensive literature review that includes thorough reference to scientific evidence. **B Good quality:** Reasonably consistent results; sufficient sample size for the study design; some control; fairly definitive conclusions; reasonably consistent recommendations based on fairly comprehensive literature review that includes some reference to scientific evidence. **C Low quality:** Little evidence with inconsistent results; insufficient sample size for the study design; conclusions cannot be drawn.
	Record findings that help answer the EBP question on page **1**

Appendix E: Research Evidence Appraisal Tool

Section I: QuaNtitative Appraisal (continued)

B Is this a summary of multiple sources of research evidence?
☐ Yes → Continue to decision tree
☐ No → Use the Nonresearch Evidence Appraisal tool (Appendix F)

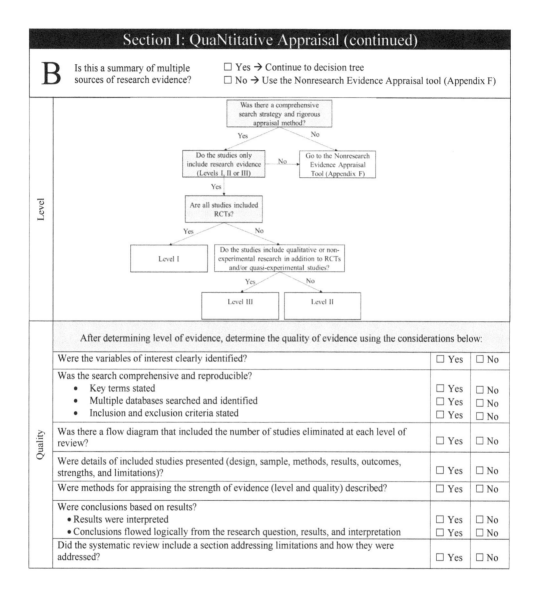

After determining level of evidence, determine the quality of evidence using the considerations below:

Were the variables of interest clearly identified?	☐ Yes	☐ No
Was the search comprehensive and reproducible? • Key terms stated • Multiple databases searched and identified • Inclusion and exclusion criteria stated	☐ Yes ☐ Yes ☐ Yes	☐ No ☐ No ☐ No
Was there a flow diagram that included the number of studies eliminated at each level of review?	☐ Yes	☐ No
Were details of included studies presented (design, sample, methods, results, outcomes, strengths, and limitations)?	☐ Yes	☐ No
Were methods for appraising the strength of evidence (level and quality) described?	☐ Yes	☐ No
Were conclusions based on results? • Results were interpreted • Conclusions flowed logically from the research question, results, and interpretation	☐ Yes ☐ Yes	☐ No ☐ No
Did the systematic review include a section addressing limitations and how they were addressed?	☐ Yes	☐ No

©2022 Johns Hopkins Health System/Johns Hopkins School of Nursing

Section I: QuaNtitative Appraisal (continued)

Circle the appropriate quality rating below:

Quality

A High quality: Topic clearly defined, literature search methods are clear and appropriate, literature thoroughly appraised and synthesized, recommendations consistent with findings, definitive conclusions can be drawn..

B Good quality: Topic defined, literature search methods are clear and appropriate, literature appraised and reasonably synthesized, recommendations consistent with findings, fairly definitive conclusions can be drawn

C Low quality: Topic not well defined, search methods lack clarity, may or may not be appropriate, literature appraisal and synthesis insufficient, recommendations inconsistent with findings, conclusions cannot be drawn.

Record findings that help answer the EBP question on page 1

Section II: QuaLitative Appraisal

A. Is this a report of a single research study?

☐ Yes → This is Level III evidence
☐ No → Go to Section II: B

After determining level of evidence, determine the quality of evidence using the considerations below:

Quality		Yes	No
	Was there a clearly identifiable and articulated: • Purpose? • Research question? • Justification for design and/or theoretical framework used?	☐ Yes ☐ Yes ☐ Yes	☐ No ☐ No ☐ No
	Do participants have knowledge of the subject the researchers are trying to explore?	☐ Yes	☐ No
	Were characteristics of study participants described?	☐ Yes	☐ No
	Was a verification process used in every step of data analysis (e.g., triangulation, response validation, independent double check, member checking)? (Credibility)	☐ Yes	☐ No
	Does the researcher provide sufficient documentation of their thinking, decisions, and methods related to the study allowing the reader to follow their decision-making (e.g., how themes and categories were formulated)? (Confirmability)	☐ Yes	☐ No
	Does the researcher provide an accurate and rich description of context to aid in the assessment of the extent to which the findings can be transferred to other settings (Transferability)?	☐ Yes	☐ No
	Does the researcher acknowledge and/or address their own role and potential influence during data collection?	☐ Yes	☐ No
	Was sampling adequate, as evidenced by achieving data saturation?	☐ Yes	☐ No
	Does the researcher provide illustrations from the data? • If yes, do the provided illustrations support conclusions?	☐ Yes ☐ Yes	☐ No ☐ No
	Is there congruency between the findings and the data?	☐ Yes	☐ No
	Is there congruency between the research methodology and: • The research question(s) • The methods to collect data • The interpretation of results	☐ Yes ☐ Yes ☐ Yes	☐ No ☐ No ☐ No
	Are discussion and conclusions congruent with the purpose and objectives, and supported by literature?	☐ Yes	☐ No
	Are conclusions drawn based on the data collected (e.g., the product of the observations or interviews)?	☐ Yes	☐ No

©2022 Johns Hopkins Health System/Johns Hopkins School of Nursing

Section II: QuaLitative Appraisal (continued)

Circle the appropriate quality rating below:

A/B High/Good Quality: The report discusses efforts to enhance or evaluate the quality of the data and the overall inquiry in sufficient detail; it describes the specific techniques used to enhance the quality of the inquiry.

Evidence of at least half or all the following is found in the report:

- *Transparency*: Describes how information was documented to justify decisions, how data were reviewed by others, and how themes and categories were formulated.
- *Diligence*: Reads and rereads data to check interpretations; seeks opportunity to find multiple sources to corroborate evidence.
- *Verification*: The process of checking, confirming, and ensuring methodologic coherence.
- *Self-reflection* and *self-scrutiny*: Being continuously aware of how a researcher's experiences, background, or prejudices might shape and bias analysis and interpretations.
- *Participant-driven inquiry*: Participants shape the scope and breadth of questions; analysis and interpretation give voice to those who participated.
- *Insightful interpretation*: Data and knowledge are linked in meaningful ways to relevant literature.

C Low quality: Lack of clarity and coherence of reporting, lack of transparency in reporting methods; poor interpretation of data and offers little insight into the phenomena of interest; few, if any, of the features listed for high/good quality.

Record findings that help answer the EBP question on page **1**

Section II: QuaLitative Appraisal

B — Is this a summary of multiple sources of qualitative research evidence with a comprehensive search strategy and rigorous appraisal method (Meta-synthesis)?

☐ Yes → This is Level III evidence
☐ No → Use the Nonresearch Evidence Appraisal tool (Appendix F)

After determining level of evidence, determine the quality of evidence using the considerations below:

Quality consideration		
Was the aim of the review clearly stated?	☐ Yes	☐ No
Were the search strategy and criteria for selecting primary studies clearly defined?	☐ Yes	☐ No
Was there a description of a systematic and thorough process for how data were analyzed?	☐ Yes	☐ No
• Were methods described for comparing findings from each study?	☐ Yes	☐ No
• Were methods described for interpreting data?	☐ Yes	☐ No
• Was sufficient data presented to support the interpretations?	☐ Yes	☐ No
Did synthesis reflect: • New insights? • Discovery of essential features of the phenomena? • A fuller understanding of the phenomena?	☐ Yes ☐ Yes ☐ Yes	☐ No ☐ No ☐ No
Are findings clearly linked to and match the data?	☐ Yes	☐ No
Are findings connected to the purpose, data collection, and analysis?	☐ Yes	☐ No
Are discussion and conclusions connected to the purpose, objectives, and (if possible) supported by literature?	☐ Yes	☐ No
Did authors describe clearly how they arrived at the interpretation of the findings?	☐ Yes	☐ No

Circle the appropriate quality rating below:

High quality: Topic and aim of the review are clearly stated. Literature search methods are clear and appropriate. Data analysis well-described. Literature thoroughly synthesized to generate deeper understanding. Findings thoroughly linked to data analysis. Definitive conclusions can be drawn.

Good Quality: Topic and aim of the review clearly stated. Literature search methods are adequate. Data analysis described. Literature reasonably synthesized to generate deeper understanding. Findings linked to data analysis. Fairly definitive conclusions can be drawn.

Low Quality: Topic and aim of review not well defined. Literature search methods lack clarity and may or may not be appropriate. Literature synthesis insufficient. Findings not sufficiently linked to data analysis. Definitive conclusions cannot be drawn.

Record findings that help answer the EBP question on page 1

©2022 Johns Hopkins Health System/Johns Hopkins School of Nursing

Section III: Mixed Methods Appraisal

You will need to appraise both parts of the study independently before appraising the study as a whole. Evaluate the quaNtitative part of the study using Section IA (single research study) or Section IIB (multiple research studies). Evaluate the qualitative part of the studying using Section IIA (single research study) or Section IIB (multiple research studies, then return here to complete appraisal.

		Level	Quality
Level	QuaNtitative Portion		
	QuaLitative Portion		

Level

The level of mixed methods evidence is based on the sequence of data collection for a single research study. QuaNtitative data collection followed by quaLitative (explanatory design) is based on the level of the quaNtitative portion. All other designs (exploratory, convergent, or multiphasic) are Level III evidence.

Explanatory sequential designs collected quantitative data first, followed by qualitative.
Exploratory sequential designs collect qualitative data first, followed by quantitative.
Convergent parallel designs collect quantitative and qualitative data at the same time.
Multiphasic designs collect qualitative and quantitative data over more than one phase.

A summary of multiple QuaNtitative and QuaLitative studies is a mixed studies review and is Level III evidence.

Quality

After determining the level of evidence, determine the quality of evidence using the considerations below:

Was the mixed-methods design appropriate to address the research question? ☐ Yes ☐ No

Circle the appropriate quality rating below:

A High quality: Contains high to good quality quaNtitative and quaLitative study components; highly relevant study design; relevant integration of data or results; and careful consideration of the limitations of the chosen approach.

B Good quality: Contains good-quality quaNtitative and quaLitative study components; relevant study design; moderately relevant integration of data or results; and some discussion of limitations of integration.

C Low quality: Contains good to low quality quaNtitative and quaLitative study components; study design not relevant to research questions or objectives; poorly integrated data or results; and no consideration of limits of integration.

Record findings that help answer the EBP question on page **1**

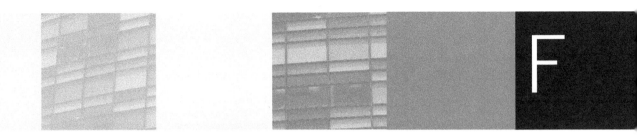

Nonresearch Evidence Appraisal Tool

Appendix F: Nonresearch Evidence Appraisal Tool

Does this evidence answer the EBP question?	☐ Yes → Continue appraisal ☐ No → STOP, do not continue evidence appraisal

Article Summary Information

Article Title:

Author(s):	Number:
Population, size, and setting:	Publication date:

Complete after appraisal:

Evidence level and quality rating:

Study findings that help answer the EBP question:

Article Appraisal Workflow

	Is this evidence:	This is…
Level	☐ A **clinical practice guideline** or a **consensus/position statement**?	**Level IV** evidence, go to **Section I: Level IV Appraisal** to determine quality
	☐ A **literature review** or **integrative review**?	**Level V** evidence, go to **Section II, A: Level V Appraisal** to determine quality
	☐ An **expert opinion**?	**Level V** evidence, go to **Section II, B: Level V Appraisal** to determine quality
	☐ **Case report**?	**Level V** evidence, go to **Section II, C: Level V Appraisal** to determine quality
	☐ An **organizational experience** (including **quality improvement**, **financial** or **program evaluations**)?	**Level V** evidence, go to **Section II, D: Level V Appraisal** to determine quality
	☐ **Community standard, clinician experience,** or **consumer preference?**	**Level V** evidence, go to **Section II, E: Level V Appraisal** to determine quality

©2022 Johns Hopkins Health System/Johns Hopkins School of Nursing

Section I: Level IV Appraisal

Select the type of Level IV evidence

☐ **Clinical practice guidelines** (systematically developed recommendations from nationally recognized experts based on research evidence or expert consensus panel)

☐ **Consensus or position statement** (systematically developed recommendations, based on research and nationally recognized expert opinion, that guide members of a professional organization in decision-making for an issue of concern)

After selecting the type of Level IV evidence, determine the quality of evidence using the considerations below:

Are the types of evidence included identified?	☐ Yes	☐ No
Were appropriate stakeholders involved in the development of recommendations?	☐ Yes	☐ No
Are groups to which recommendations apply and do not apply clearly defined?	☐ Yes	☐ No
Does each recommendation have an identified level of evidence stated?	☐ Yes	☐ No
Are recommendations clear?	☐ Yes	☐ No

Circle the appropriate quality rating below:

A High quality: Material officially sponsored by a professional, public, or private organization or a government agency; documentation of a systematic literature search strategy; consistent results with sufficient numbers of well-designed studies; criteria-based evaluation of overall scientific strength and quality of included studies and definitive conclusions; national expertise clearly evident; developed or revised within the past five years.

B Good quality: Material officially sponsored by a professional, public, or private organization or a government agency; reasonably thorough and appropriate systematic literature search strategy; reasonably consistent results, sufficient numbers of well-designed studies; evaluation of strengths and limitations of included studies with fairly definitive conclusions; national expertise clearly evident; developed or revised within the past five years.

C Low quality: Material not sponsored by an official organization or agency; undefined, poorly defined, or limited literature search strategy; no evaluation of strengths and limitations of included studies; insufficient evidence with inconsistent results; conclusions cannot be drawn; not revised within the past five years.

Record findings that help answer the EBP question on page 1

Section II: Level V Quality Appraisal

A Select the type of article:

☐ **Literature review** (summary of selected published literature including scientific and nonscientific, such as reports of organizational experience and opinions of experts)

☐ **Integrative review** (summary of research evidence and theoretical literature; analyzes, compares themes, notes gaps in the selected literature)

After selecting the type of Level V evidence, determine the quality of evidence using the considerations below:		
Is subject matter to be reviewed clearly stated?	☐ Yes	☐ No
Is literature relevant and up-to-date (most sources are within the past five years or classic)?	☐ Yes	☐ No
Of the literature reviewed, is there a meaningful analysis of the conclusions across the articles included in the review?	☐ Yes	☐ No
Are gaps in the literature identified?	☐ Yes	☐ No
Are recommendations made for future practice or study?	☐ Yes	☐ No

Circle the appropriate quality rating below:

A High quality: Expertise is clearly evident, draws definitive conclusions, and provides scientific rationale; thought leader in the field.

B Good quality: Expertise appears to be credible, draws fairly definitive conclusions, and provides logical argument for opinions.

C Low quality: Expertise is not discernable or is dubious; conclusions cannot be drawn.

Record findings that help answer the EBP question on page **1**

Section II: Level V Quality Appraisal (continued)

B Select the type of article:

☐ **Expert opinion** (opinion of one or more individuals based on clinical expertise)

<table>
<tr><td colspan="3">After selecting the type of Level V evidence, determine the quality of evidence using the considerations below:</td></tr>
<tr><td>Does the author have relevant education and training?</td><td>☐ Yes</td><td>☐ No</td></tr>
<tr><td>Do they have relevant professional and academic affiliations?</td><td>☐ Yes</td><td>☐ No</td></tr>
<tr><td>Have they previously published in the area of interest?</td><td>☐ Yes</td><td>☐ No</td></tr>
<tr><td>Have they been recognized by state, regional, national, or international groups for their expertise?</td><td>☐ Yes</td><td>☐ No</td></tr>
<tr><td>Are their publications well cited by others?</td><td>☐ Yes</td><td>☐ No</td></tr>
<tr><td colspan="3" align="center">*A web search can provide information about expertise*</td></tr>
<tr><td colspan="3" align="center">Circle the appropriate quality rating below:</td></tr>
<tr><td colspan="3">

A High quality: Expertise is clearly evident, draws definitive conclusions, and provides scientific rationale; thought leader in the field.

B Good quality: Expertise appears to be credible, draws fairly definitive conclusions, and provides logical argument for opinions.

C Low quality: Expertise is not discernable or is dubious; conclusions cannot be drawn.
</td></tr>
<tr><td colspan="3" align="center">Record findings that help answer the EBP question on page 1</td></tr>
</table>

©2022 Johns Hopkins Health System/Johns Hopkins School of Nursing

Section II: Level V Quality Appraisal (continued)

C Select the type of article:

☐ **Case report** (an in-depth look at a person or group or another social unit)

<table>
<tr><td rowspan="6">Quality</td><td colspan="3">After selecting the type of Level V evidence, determine the quality of evidence using the considerations below:</td></tr>
<tr><td>Is the purpose of the case report clearly stated?</td><td>☐ Yes</td><td>☐ No</td></tr>
<tr><td>Is the case report clearly presented?</td><td>☐ Yes</td><td>☐ No</td></tr>
<tr><td>Are the findings of the case report supported by relevant theory or research?</td><td>☐ Yes</td><td>☐ No</td></tr>
<tr><td>Are the recommendations clearly stated and linked to the findings?</td><td>☐ Yes</td><td>☐ No</td></tr>
<tr><td colspan="3">Circle the appropriate quality rating below:

A High quality: Expertise is clearly evident, draws definitive conclusions, and provides scientific rationale; thought leader in the field.

B Good quality: Expertise appears to be credible, draws fairly definitive conclusions, and provides logical argument for opinions.

C Low quality: Expertise is not discernable or is dubious; conclusions cannot be drawn.</td></tr>
<tr><td colspan="3" align="center">Record findings that help answer the EBP question on page **1**</td></tr>
</table>

©2022 Johns Hopkins Health System/Johns Hopkins School of Nursing

Section II: Level V Quality Appraisal (continued)

D Select the type of article:

☐ **Quality improvement** (cyclical method to examine workflows, processes, or systems within a specific organization)

☐ **Financial evaluation** (economic evaluation that applies analytic techniques to identify, measure, and compare the cost and outcomes of two or more alternative programs or interventions)

☐ **Program evaluation** (systematic assessment of the processes and/or outcomes of a program; can involve both quaNtitative and quaLitative methods)

After selecting the type of Level V evidence, determine the quality of evidence using the considerations below:			
Was the aim of the project clearly stated?	☐ Yes	☐ No	
Was a formal QI method used for conducting or reporting the project (e.g., PDSA, SQUIRE 2.0)?	☐ Yes	☐ No	
Was the method fully described?	☐ Yes	☐ No	
Were process or outcome measures identified?	☐ Yes	☐ No	
Were results fully described?	☐ Yes	☐ No	
Was interpretation clear and appropriate?	☐ Yes	☐ No	
Are components of cost/benefit or cost effectiveness data described?	☐ Yes	☐ No	☐ N/A

Circle the appropriate quality rating below:

A High quality: Clear aims and objectives; consistent results across multiple settings; formal quality improvement or financial evaluation methods used; definitive conclusions; consistent recommendations with thorough reference to scientific evidence.

B Good quality: Clear aims and objectives; formal quality improvement or financial evaluation methods used; consistent results in a single setting; reasonably consistent recommendations with some reference to scientific evidence.

C Low quality: Unclear or missing aims and objectives; inconsistent results; poorly defined quality improvement/financial analysis method; recommendations cannot be made.

Record findings that help answer the EBP question on page **1**

Section II: Level V Quality Appraisal (continued)

E Select the type of article:

- ☐ **Community standard** (current practice for comparable settings in the community)
- ☐ **Clinician experience** (knowledge gained through practice experience from the clinician perspective)
- ☐ **Consumer preference** (knowledge gained through life experience from the patient perspective)

Record the sources of information and the number of sources:

Quality

After selecting the type of Level V evidence, determine the quality of evidence using the considerations below:

Source of information has credible experience	☐ Yes	☐ No	☐ N/A
Opinions are clearly stated	☐ Yes	☐ No	☐ N/A
Evidence obtained is consistent	☐ Yes	☐ No	☐ N/A

Circle the appropriate quality rating below:

A High quality: Expertise is clearly evident, draws definitive conclusions, and provides scientific rationale; thought leader in the field.

B Good quality: Expertise appears to be credible, draws fairly definitive conclusions, and provides logical argument for opinions.

C Low quality: Expertise is not discernable or is dubious; conclusions cannot be drawn.

Record findings that help answer the EBP question on page 1

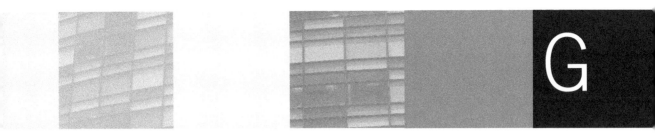

Individual Evidence Summary Tool

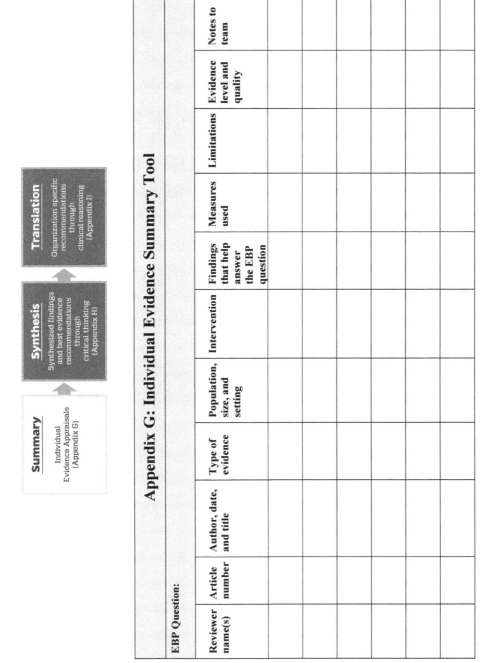

Appendix G: Individual Evidence Summary Tool

EBP Question:

Reviewer name(s)	Article number	Author, date, and title	Type of evidence	Population, size, and setting	Intervention	Findings that help answer the EBP question	Measures used	Limitations	Evidence level and quality	Notes to team

Directions for use of the Individual Evidence Summary Tool

Purpose: Use this form to document and collate the results of the review and appraisal of each piece of evidence in preparation for evidence synthesis. The table headers indicate important elements of each article that will contribute to the synthesis process. The data in each cell should be complete enough that the other team members are able to gather all relevant information related to the evidence without having to go to each source article.

> **See Chapter 11, Lessons from Practice, for examples of completed tools.**

Reviewer name(s):
Record the member(s) of the team who are providing the information for each article. This will provide tracking if there are follow-up items or additional questions on an individual piece of evidence.

Article number:
Assign a number to each piece of evidence included in the table. This organizes the individual evidence summary and provides an easy way to reference articles.

Author, date, and title:
Record the last name of the first author of the article, the publication/communication date, and the title. This will help track articles throughout the literature search, screening, and review process. It is also helpful when someone has authored more than one publication included in the review.

Type of evidence:
Indicate the type of evidence for each source. This should be descriptive of the study or project design (e.g., randomized control trial, meta-analysis, mixed methods, qualitative, systematic review, case study, literature review) and not simply the level on the evidence hierarchy.

©2022 Johns Hopkins Health System/Johns Hopkins School of Nursing

Population, size, and setting:

For research evidence, provide a quick view of the population, number of participants, and study location. For non-research evidence population refers to target audience, patient population, or profession. Non-research evidence may or may not have a sample size and/or location as found with research evidence.

Intervention:

Record the intervention(s) implemented or discussed in the article. This should relate to the intervention or comparison elements of your PICO question.

Findings that help answer the EBP question:

List findings from the article that directly answer the EBP question. These should be succinct statements that provide enough information that the reader does not need to return to the original article. Avoid directly copying and pasting from the article.

Measures used:

These are the measures and/or instruments (e.g., counts, rates, satisfaction surveys, validated tools, subscales) the authors used to determine the answer to the research question or the effectiveness of their intervention. Consider these measures as identified in the evidence for collection during implementation of the EBP team's project.

Limitations:

Provide the limitations of the evidence—both as listed by the authors as well as your assessment of any flaws or drawbacks. Consider the methodology, quality of reporting, and generalizability to the population of interest. Limitations should be apparent from the team's appraisals using the Research and Non-Research Evidence Appraisal Tools (Appendices E and F). It can be helpful to consider the reasons an article did not receive a "high" quality rating because these reasons are limitations identified by the team.

Evidence level and quality:

Using the Research and Non-Research Evidence Appraisal tools (Appendices E and F), record the level (I-V) and quality (A, B or C) of the evidence. When possible, at least two reviewers should determine the level and quality.

Notes to team:

The team uses this section to keep track of items important to the EBP process not captured elsewhere on this tool. Consider items that will be helpful to have easy reference to when conducting the evidence synthesis.

©2022 Johns Hopkins Health System/Johns Hopkins School of Nursing

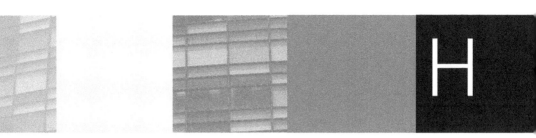

Synthesis and Recommendations Tool

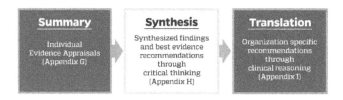

Appendix H: Synthesis and Recommendations Tools

EBP Question:

Level	Strength — Overall Quality Rating (Strong, good, or low)	Number of Sources (Quantity)	Synthesized Findings With Article Number(s) (This is *not* a simple restating of information from each individual evidence summary—see directions)
Level I ▪ Experimental studies			
Level II ▪ Quasi-experimental studies			
Level III ▪ Nonexperimental, including qualitative studies			
Level IV ▪ Clinical practice guidelines or consensus panels			
Level V ▪ Literature reviews, QI, case reports, expert opinion			

©2022 Johns Hopkins Health System/Johns Hopkins School of Nursing

Appendix H: Synthesis and Recommendations Tool

Where does the evidence show consistency?

Where does the evidence show inconsistency?

Best evidence recommendations (taking into consideration quantity, consistency, and strength of the evidence):

Based on your synthesis, select the statement that best describes the overall characteristics of the body of evidence?

☐ **Strong & compelling evidence, consistent results →** Recommendations are reliable; evaluate for organizational translation.

☐ **Good evidence & consistent results →** Recommendations may be reliable; evaluate for risk and organizational translation.

☐ **Good evidence but conflicting results →** Unable to establish best practice based on current evidence; evaluate risk, consider further investigation for new evidence, develop a research study, or discontinue the project.

☐ **Little or no evidence →** Unable to establish best practice based on current evidence; consider further investigation for new evidence, develop a research study, or discontinue the project.

©2022 Johns Hopkins Health System/Johns Hopkins School of Nursing

Directions for use of the Synthesis and Recommendations Tool

Purpose:

> See Chapter 11, Lessons from Practice, for examples of completed tools.

This tool guides the EBP team through the process of synthesizing the pertinent findings from the Individual Evidence Summary (Appendix G), sorted by evidence level, to create an overall picture of the body of the evidence related to the PICO question. The synthesis process uses quantity, strength (level and quality), and consistency to generate best evidence recommendations for potential translation.

Overall quality rating and total number of sources:

Record the overall quality rating and the number of sources for each level (strong, good, or low), ensuring agreement among the team members.

Synthesized findings:

This section captures key findings that answer the EBP question. Using the questions below, generate a comprehensive synthesis by combining the different pieces of evidence in the form of succinct statements that enhance the team's knowledge and generate new insights, perspectives, and understandings into a greater whole. The following questions can help guide the team's discussion of the evidence:

- How can the evidence in each of the levels be organized to produce a more comprehensive understanding of the big picture?
- What themes do you notice?
- What elements of the intervention/setting/sample seem to influence the outcome?
- What are the important takeaways?

Avoid repeating content and/or copying and pasting directly from the Individual Evidence Summary Tool. Record the article number(s) used to generate each synthesis statement to make the source of findings easy to identify.

Using this synthesis tool requires not only the critical thinking of the whole team, but also group discussion and consensus building. The team reviews the individual evidence summary of high- and good-quality articles, uses subjective and objective reasoning to look for salient themes, and evaluates information to create higher-level insights. They include and consider the strength and consistency of findings in their evaluation.

Where does the evidence show consistency/inconsistency?

EBP teams must consider how consistent the results are across studies. Do the studies tend to show the same conclusions, or are there differences? The synthesized evidence is much more compelling when most studies have the same general results or point in the same general direction. The synthesized evidence is less compelling when the results from half the studies have one indication, while the findings from the other half point in a different direction. The team should identify the points of consistency among the evidence as well as areas where inconsistency is apparent. Both factors are important to consider when developing recommendations or determining next steps.

Best evidence recommendations:

In this section, the EBP team takes into consideration all the above information related to strength, quantity, and consistency of the synthesized findings at each level to generate best practice recommendations from the evidence. Consider:

- What is the strength and quantity of studies related to a specific evidence recommendation?
- Is there a sufficient number of high-strength studies to support one recommendation over another?
- Are there any recommendations that can be ruled out based on the strength and quantity of the evidence?
- Does the team feel the evidence is of sufficient strength and quantity to be considered a best evidence recommendation?

Recommendations should be succinct statements that distill the synthesized evidence into an answer to the EBP question. The team bases these recommendations on the evidence and does not yet consider their specific setting. Translating the recommendations into action steps within the team's organization occurs in the next step (Translation and Action Planning Tool, Appendix I).

Based on the synthesis, which statement represents the overall body of the evidence?

Choose the statement that best reflects the strength and congruence of the findings. This determination will help the team to decide next steps in the translation process.

When evidence is *strong* (includes multiple high-quality studies of Level I and Level II evidence), compelling, and consistent, EBP teams can have greater confidence in best practice recommendations and should begin organizational translation

When most of the evidence is *good* (high-quality Level II and Level III) *and consistent* or *good but conflicting*, the team should proceed cautiously in making practice changes. In this instance, translation typically includes evaluating risk and careful consideration for organizational translation.

The team makes practice changes primarily when evidence exists that is of high to good strength. Never make practice changes on *little to no evidence* (low-quality evidence at any level or Level IV or Level V evidence alone). Nonetheless, teams have a variety of options for actions that include, but are not limited to, creating awareness campaigns, conducting informational and educational updates, monitoring evidence sources for new information, and designing research studies.

The exact quantity of sources needed to determine the strength of the evidence is subjective and depends on many factors, including the topic and amount of available literature. The EBP team should discuss what they consider sufficient given their knowledge of the problem, literature, and setting

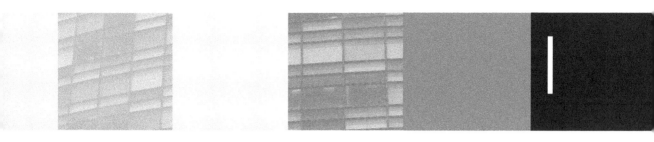

Translation and Action Planning Tool

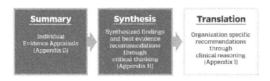

Appendix I: Translation and Action Planning Tool

Translation

Select the statement that best describes the overall characteristics of the body of evidence from the team's synthesis and recommendations (Appendix H):

☐ Strong & compelling evidence, consistent results ☐ Good but conflicting evidence
☐ Good & consistent evidence ☒ Little or no evidence

What is the level of safety risk associated with the intervention?

☐ High   ☐ Low

Translation Assessment Flowchart:

Start Here → Strong, compelling evidence. Consistent results? — YES → Change is indicated

NO ↓

Good and consistent evidence? — YES → What is the level of risk or potential for harm if implemented?
— LOW → Consider pilot of change or further investigation
— HIGH → No indication for practice change, monitor for new evidence, develop a research study or discontinue project

NO ↓

Good but conflicting evidence? — YES ↑

NO ↓

Little or no evidence? — YES →

Based on the Translation Assessment, select the course of action:

☐ Change is indicated (system or process improvement, or practice), go to Section I

☐ Consider a pilot of the change or further investigation for new evidence, go to Section I.

☐ No indication for change or consider further investigation for new evidence, develop a research study or discontinue project, go to Section II.

Section I: If change is indicated, generate organization-specific recommendations by assessing the best-evidence recommendations for feasibility, fit, and acceptability:	
Feasibility Extent to which the team evaluates and believes that the change is low risk, doable, and can be successfully implemented within a given organization or setting.	☐ The change is low risk. ☐ Few, if any, barriers identified, and the time, effort, and resources to overcome them is reasonable. ☐ Sponsors or leaders share their point of view, endorse and support the change
Fit Compatibility of a change with end user workflow and consumer expectations; and/or the perceived relevance of the change in addressing the problem and in answering the PICO question within a given practice setting.	☐ The change aligns with unit and/or departmental priorities. ☐ The change is suitable and seems like a good match with end-user workflow. ☐ The change is applicable to the problem and answers the PICO question.
Acceptability Extent to which stakeholders and organizational leadership perceive the change to be agreeable, palatable, satisfactory, and reasonable.	☐ The change aligns with organizational priorities. ☐ The change meets the approval of stakeholders and organizational leadership. ☐ Stakeholders and leaders like and welcome the change and find it appealing.
Organization-specific recommendations:	
Section II: When a change or pilot is not indicated, what, if any, next steps does the EBP team recommend?	

©2022 Johns Hopkins Health System/Johns Hopkins School of Nursing

Action Planning

Complete the following activities to ensure successful implementation:

- ❏ Secure a project leader
- ❏ Identify change champions
- ❏ Consider whether translation activities require different or additional members
- ❏ Identify objectives and related tasks
- ❏ Determine dates to complete tasks
- ❏ Identify observable pre and post measures

Identify strengths that can be leveraged to overcome barriers to ensure the success of the change:

Resources or Strengths	Barriers	Plan to Overcome Barriers by Leveraging Strengths as Appropriate

Which of the following will be affected by this change? (*Select all that apply*)

☐ Electronic health record   ☐ Workflow   ☐ Policies and/or procedures   ☐ Other_____

Identify and secure the resources and/or funding required for translation and implementation: (*Check all that apply*)

☐ Personnel costs   ☐ Content or external experts
☐ Supplies/equipment   ☐ Dissemination costs (conference costs, travel)
☐ Technology   ☐ Other: _____
☐ Education or further training

Outcomes Measurement Plan					
What is/are the goal(s) of the project?				Desired completion date:	
How will you know if you are successful?	**Types of Outcomes**		**Selected Metrics**	**Source**	**Frequency**
	☐ **Clinical** (e.g., vital signs, infection rates, fall rates, adverse events)				
	☐ **Functional** (e.g., activities of daily living, quality of life, self-medication administration)				
	☐ **Perceptual** (e.g., satisfaction, care experience, timeliness of response)				
	☐ **Process/Intervention** (e.g., care coordination, immunization, bereavement support)				
	☐ **Organization/Unit-Based** (e.g., staffing levels, length of stay, readmissions)				
Work Breakdown Structure					
High Level Deliverable	**Associated Tasks and Sub-Tasks**		**Start Date**	**End Date**	**Responsible Party**

©2022 Johns Hopkins Health System/Johns Hopkins School of Nursing

Directions for use of the Translation and Action Planning Tool

Purpose:

> See Chapter 11, Lessons from Practice, for examples of completed tools.

This tool guides the EBP team through the process of analyzing the best-evidence recommendations for translation into the team's specific setting. The translation process considers the strength, consistency, risk, fit, and acceptability of the best-evidence recommendations. The team uses both critical thinking and clinical reasoning to generate site-specific recommendations.

Translation Section

What is the overall state of the evidence from the team's synthesis and recommendations (Appendix H)?

Consult the Synthesis and Recommendations Tool (Appendix H) and record the group's determination regarding the overall description of the state of the evidence.

What is the level of safety risk associated with the intervention?

Different interventions carry different levels and types of risks. As a group, the EBP team should discuss the potential for harm to patients, staff, or the community associated with the best-evidence recommendations. While other factors, such as monetary risks, may be important, this question refers specifically to dangers related to safety. Select "high" or "low" from the list of options.

Based on the Translation Assessment Flowchart, select the course of action:

Use the Translation Assessment Flowchart to determine next steps for potential translation. Select the course of action indicated from the flowchart.

If change is indicated, generate organization-specific recommendations by assessing the best-evidence recommendations for feasibility, fit, and acceptability:

The EBP team uses the prompts to assess the feasibility, fit, and acceptability of the best-evidence recommendations to determine the likelihood of successful implementation and to generate recommendations specific to their setting. Feasibility, fit, and acceptability take into account the practice setting's characteristics such as culture, norms, beliefs, structures, priorities, workflow, and resources. Depending on the setting, organization-specific recommendations may mirror the best-evidence recommendations, differ significantly, or be deemed inappropriate for implementation by the organization. List recommendations for the organization in the space provided in a series of actionable and concise statements. If they differ from the best-evidence recommendations, include information for feasibility, fit, and acceptability related changes.

Feasibility: Extent to which the team evaluates and believes that the change is low risk, doable, and can be successfully implemented within a given organization or setting.

Fit: Compatibility of a change with end-user workflow and consumer expectations; and/or the perceived relevance of the change in addressing the problem and in answering the PICO question within a given practice setting.

Acceptability: Extent to which stakeholders and organizational leadership perceive the change to be agreeable, palatable, satisfactory, and reasonable.

When a change or pilot is not undertaken, what, if any, next steps does the EBP team recommend?

If the team cannot recommend a change or pilot, record future directions for the project. This might include proposing a research study, waiting until more evidence becomes available, or discontinuing the project altogether.

Action Planning Section

Complete the following activities to ensure successful translation:

This list provides steps to assist the team with completing the practice change(s) associated with their EBP project.

Identify strengths that can be leveraged to overcome barriers to ensure the success of the change:

This analysis allows teams to identify barriers to implementation and potentially mitigate them using inherent strengths and resources. You may find specific challenges that will likely impact the ability to deliver on the action plan. Though these obstacles can get in the way, knowing about them up front is helpful so that you can engage support and create a plan to move forward.

Consider whether or how this change will impact workflows and processes:

This section assists the team in considering downstream effects of a change. For example, will adjustments need to be made to the electronic medical record to accommodate the change, or will this change impact the workflow of any other staff who have not been considered?

Identify and secure the resources and/or funding required for translation and implementation:

Use this as a guide to consider and plan for financial obligations that may be part of the rollout.

Outcomes Measurement Plan

What is/are the goal(s) of the project?

Record what the team hopes to accomplish by implementing the change(s). These can be high level statements used to inform the measurement plan and implementation.

Desired completion date:

Record when the team plans to complete the first stage of the project. The team determines the anticipated implementation date and the outcomes data that will be needed to evaluate success. This can be updated throughout implementation to reflect adjustments to the timeline.

How will you know if you are successful?

Use this table to agree upon outcomes the team will collect and analyze to monitor the success of the project. There are different aspects to practice change, and frequently different measures are used to monitor uptake, attitudes, and outcomes. Select as many as the team feels are necessary to gain an accurate picture of ongoing impact. Record the specific metric(s) the team will measure within the outcome categories, how the metrics will be obtained, and how often. Outcomes can be added or changed as the review of the literature is completed and the translation planning begins.

Metrics let you know whether the change was successful. They have a numerator and a denominator and are typically expressed as rates or percentages. For example, a metric for the measure falls-with-injury would be the number of falls with injury (numerator) divided by 1,000 patient days (denominator). Other examples of metrics include the number of direct care RNs (numerator) on a unit divided by the total number of direct care staff (denominator); or the number of medication errors divided by 1,000 orders.

Work Breakdown Structure:

A Work Breakdown Structure (WBS) is a deliverable-oriented prioritized list of the steps needed to accomplish the project objectives and create the required deliverables.

Consider all the categories of work (high level deliverables) necessary to implement this change. What tasks must be accomplished first for each deliverable in order to move forward? When must they be completed to stay on track? For example, if a high level deliverable is needed to implement a protocol, list all tasks to accomplish it. Record when the team must begin and complete the task, and which member(s) are responsible. If possible, list a specific person or role to create ownership of work.

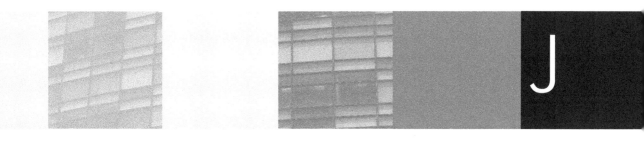

Publication Guide

Appendix J: Publication Guide

Template for Publishing an Evidence-Based Practice Project

Title and Abstract
Title: Identifies the report/project as an evidence-based project
Abstract: Provide a summary which includes, as applicable: the rationale for the EBP project, with EBP question, literature search and appraisal methods, results, best-evidence synthesis, and organizational translation recommendations.

Introduction	
Appendix B	**Rationale for the EBP Project**: Describe the problem, internal data to validate the problem, the problem's importance, risks of not addressing the problem, and the current practice.
	Available Knowledge: Include what is currently known about the problem from the literature to create a broad view (e.g., organizationally, nationally, globally).
	EBP Question: Provide the EBP question being addressed using the PICO format.

Methods	
Appendix B	**Information Sources**: Describe the sources (e.g., databases, standards, clinical practice guidelines, organizational data, evidence-based professional organization position statements, consensus studies) used in the evidence search.
	Search Methods: Describe the inclusion and exclusion criteria, date ranges, and rationale for search strategy limits.
	Keywords: List the keywords, phrases, or search concepts used for the literature search.
	Article Screening: Describe the process for title, abstract, and full text screening of literature search results.

Appendix J: Publication Guide   335

	Data Collection and Article Appraisal Process: Explain the process for completing the article appraisal process, including the model used (Johns Hopkins Evidence-Based Model and Guidelines), the number of reviewers, elements collected in the individual evidence summary tool, and how the team resolved discrepancies/reached consensus.
	Synthesis, Recommendations, and Translation Process: Describe the process used to synthesize the evidence, generate best-evidence recommendations, and translate this to the team's setting.

	Results
	Study Selection: Provide the number of articles screened by the EBP team, including the final number of articles included in the synthesis and recommendations. Consider using a flow diagram.
Appendix G	**Study Characteristics**: Provide the relevant information from the individual evidence summary for all included articles (e.g., author, type of evidence, population size and setting, intervention, findings that answer the EBP question, measures used, limitations, and level and quality rating) in table format.
	Findings of Individual Studies: Consider the value of including additional elements of interest of each study by visual display (table, figure, or chart) to provide more in-depth description and clarity.

	Discussion
Appendix H	**Synthesis of Evidence**: Synthesize the findings of the overall evidence review including the strength (level, quality), quantity, and best evidence recommendations.
	Limitations: Discuss the limitations of the project. This can include limitations of the articles within the review (e.g., low quality, small sample sizes) and limitations of the review process itself (e.g., difficulty retrieving all relevant articles).
	Conclusions: Include a brief restatement of the problem and why it is important and a broad interpretation of relevant findings—avoid summarizing key points. Show whether, or to what extent, the project succeeded in answering the PICO question and addressing the problem.

©2022 Johns Hopkins Health System/Johns Hopkins School of Nursing

	Implications
Appendix C & I	**Translation Strategies**: Describe the organization-specific recommendations and action plan, including considerations of risk, fit, feasibility, acceptability, and stakeholder engagement.
Appendix I	**Outcomes**: Identify the measure used to determine the success of any changes associated with the project. If the project has been implemented, report on relevant outcomes.

Directions for Use of the Dissemination Tool

Purpose: This template is a structured guide for writing a manuscript for publishing an evidence-based practice project. Each section above includes the aspects of the project required for developing a robust manuscript. It can also help divide the writing among team members and provides guidance on which elements of the EBP project fall under each heading (introduction, methods, results, and conclusion) without redundancy. When used, the JHEBP Model tools provide much of the information needed for a manuscript. Use the appendix references to locate the team's previous work. This template was created with reference to the SQUIRE 2.0 guidelines (Ogrinc et al., 2016), PRISMA Statement (Moher et al., 2009), and Evidence-Based Practice Process Quality Assessment Guidelines (Lee et al., 2013).

References

Lee, M. C., Johnson, K. L., Newhouse, R. P., & Warren, J. I. (2013). Evidence-based practice process quality assessment: EPQA guidelines. *Worldviews on Evidence-Based Nursing, 10*(3), 140–149. https://doi.org/10.1111/j.1741-6787.2012.00264.x

Moher, D., Liberati, A., Tetzlaff, J., Altman, D. G., & the PRISMA Group. (2009). Preferred reporting items for systematic reviews and meta-analyses: The PRISMA statement. *BMJ, 339*, b2535. https://doi.org/10.1136/bmj.b2535

Ogrinc, G., Davies, L., Goodman, D., Batalden, P. B., Davidoff, F., & Stevens, D. (2016). SQUIRE 2.0 (Standards for QUality Improvement Reporting Excellence): Revised publication guidelines from a detailed consensus process. *BMJ Quality and Safety, 25*(12), 986–992. https://doi.org/10.1136/bmjqs-2015-004411

Index

NOTE: Page references noted with a *b* are boxes; page references noted with an *f* are figures; page references noted with a *t* are tables.

A

ABIM Foundation, 32
abstracts, 117, 153
acceptability recommendations, 196–198
access to information/library services, 31
accountability, evidence-based practice (EBP) and, 8–9
accreditation, 7, 53
action items, 80, 325–332
Action Planning Tool, 271–275
action plans, 63–64
    implementing, 64, 200–201, 202
    support for, 64
    translation, 198–200
adopters
    curves, 77*f*
    five categories of, 76*b*
adoption of evidence-based practice (EBP), 17
Advisory Board Company, 182
Advisory Committee on Immunization Practices, 14
Affordable Care Act 2010, 181

Agency for Healthcare Research and Quality (AHRQ), 113, 121, 144, 144*t*, 167, 192*t*
algorithms, 165
American Association of Colleges of Nursing (AACN), 44
American Association of Respiratory Care, 46
American College of Chest Physicians (CHEST), 165
American College of Clinical Pharmacy, 46
American Nurses Association (ANA), 45, 46, 104
American Nurses Credentialing Center (ANCC), 47, 53, 211
analysis, 7. *See also* tools
    Stakeholder Analysis and Communication Tool, 252–253, 289–293
    systematic reviews with meta-analysis, 142–143, 158–159
AND operator, 108, 109, 110*t*
answerable questions, 101–102
appraisal
    articles, 225*f*
    evidence, 129 (*see also* research)
    nonresearch (*see* nonresearch)

Nonresearch Evidence Appraisal Tool, 261–265, 307–314
quality of evidence, 147–160
Research Evidence Appraisal Tool, 160, 254–260, 297–306
Appraisal of Guidelines for Research and Evaluation (AGREE) II Tool, 233
Appraisal of Guidelines Research and Evaluation (AGREE) Collaboration, 165, 166
appraisal techniques, 29
Nonresearch Evidence Appraisal Tool, 60
Research Evidence Appraisal Tool, 60
articles
appraisal, 225f
peer-reviewed journal, 213–216
searching, 235
assessments, loss, 27. *See also* evaluation
attention bias, 149t
audience, dissemination, 208
authorship, citing, 215b. *See also* writing
averages, 150

background questions, 86–90
backgrounds (for presentations), 213
barriers, overcoming, 24–25
behavior, frequency of, 139
Behavioral Measurement Database Services, 107
benefits, 5
Best Practice information sheets, 101, 106
best practices companies, 182
best qualitative, 141t
biases
searching, 100, 103
types of, 149t
validity and, 148

bodies of evidence, 165. *See also* evidence
Boolean operators, 108, 109, 110t, 168

Campaign Zero, 181
The Campbell Collaboration, 144t
capacity, building, 29–33
case-control, 138, 139t
case reports, 178–179
case studies, 141t
Centers for Disease Control and Prevention (CDC), 113, 175
Centers for Medicare & Medicaid Services (CMS), 53, 100
central tendency, measures of, 150
Centre for Reviews and Dissemination (CRD), 144t
change
champions, 200
communication, 200t
Plan-Do-Study-Act (PDSA), 64, 65
practice, 90
change-and-transition processes, 28, 33–35. *See also* transitions
change management, 17, 20
change champions, 23
definition of change, 26t
leadership participation in, 18, 22
maintenance of, 25
managing transitions, 26–27
change teams, 28
CINAHL (Cumulative Index to Nursing and Allied Health Literature), 4, 32, 100, 101, 104, 108, 224, 232, 235, 238
filters, 109
CINAHL Plus, 254
CINAHL *Subject Headings*, 104
citations, identifying, 118

citing authorship, 215*b*
clarification of problems, 56–57
clarity of teams, 78
classification systems, 121
clinical practice guidelines (CPGs), 164–167, 166*t*–167*t*
Clinical Practice Guidelines We Can Trust (IOM [2011]), 170
clinical queries (PubMed), 105
clinical questions, 82
clinical reasoning, 51–52
Clinical Trials.gov, 112
clinician experience, 179–180
Cochrane, Archibald L., 6
Cochrane Collaboration, 6, 32, 145*t*
Cochrane Database of Systematic Reviews, 106, 238
Cochrane Handbook for Systematic Reviews of Interventions, 116
Cochrane Library, 100, 101, 106, 121, 254
Cochrane Review, 91
cohorts, 138, 139*t*
collaboration
   Appraisal of Guidelines Research and Evaluation (AGREE) Collaboration, 165
   group, 50
   identifying, 75
   interprofessional, 32–33
collecting evidence, 99. *See also* evidence
Commission on Accreditation of Rehabilitation Facilities, 53
committees, structures of, 34, 35*t*
communication, 26
   change, 200*t*
   lack of, 25
   planning, 35–37
   Stakeholder Analysis and Communication Tool, 252–253, 289–293
   strategies, 209–210

community standards, 179
companies, best practices, 182
comparisons (PICO), 57, 88, 89, 90. *See also* PICO
competencies, 242
   development of, 49
   healthcare professionals (HCPs), 47*f*
   identifying, 74
Competency Domain, 32
components, 44–49
   of action plans, 198–200
   of fit recommendations, 196–198
   of inquiry, 45
   of learning, 48–49
   of manuscript submissions, 216*t*
   of practice, 45–48
   of practice setting-specific recommendations, 196
   of translation, 196–203
conclusions, 153, 154
Conduct and Utilization of Research in Nursing Project (CURN), 6
conferences, 32, 211–213
confidence intervals (CIs), 152
conflicts of interest (COIs), 166*t*, 171
connectivism, 50
consensus statements (CSs), 165
Consensus Study (IOM), 74
consistency, Heat Charts, 197, 197*f*
CONsolidated Standards of Reporting Trials (CONSORT), 170
construct validity, 147
consumer experience, 180–181
content validity, 148
control, 134
control groups, 134, 135
controlled vocabularies, 108
core competencies, 46
   development of, 49
   healthcare professionals (HCPs), 47*f*

correlational studies, 138–139
costs, 5, 7
cover letters, 216t
COVID-19, 212, 240
critical reviews, 169t
critical thinking, 51–52, 61
critiques, 24, 29. *See also* feedback
cross-cultural validity, 148
Crossing the Quality Chasm (2001), 14
cross-sectional studies, 136
cultures. *See also* environments
    building capacity, 29–33
    creating EBP, 241–243
    developing mentors, 22–23
    developing strategic plans, 21
    establishing organizational, 19–29
    implementation plans, 24
    learning, 48
    managing transitions, 26–27
    organizational, 53, 199
    overcoming barriers, 24–25
    transition strategies, 27–29
curves, adopters, 77f
cycles
    Plan-Do-Study-Act (PDSA), 64, 65, 174, 175, 191, 193–195, 227, 228
    rapid cycle quality improvement (QI), 193

D

databases, 100, 101, 254
    Behavioral Measurement Database Services, 107
    Boolean operators, 108, 109
    Cochrane Database of Systematic Reviews, 106
    creating search strategies, 107–114
    ERIC, 238
    filters, 109
    Health and Psychosocial Instruments (HaPI), 107
    literature, 32, 101
    outside of nursing literature, 106–107
    Physiotherapy Evidence Database (PEDro), 107
    PsycINFO, 106–107
    selecting, 104–106
    TRIP Medical Database, 112
decision-making, 5, 165, 201
decision trees, 92f
dependability, 78
dependent variables, 134
descriptive studies, 137–138, 145–146
design, 131–141
    correlational studies, 138–139
    descriptive studies, 137–138
    non-experimental research, 133t, 136
    poster presentations, 211, 212
    qualitative research, 140–141
    quasi-experimental research, 132t, 135–136
    single study research, 132–141
    systematic reviews, 141–146
    true experimental research, 132t, 133–135
    univariate research, 133t, 139–140
development groups, guidelines, 164, 166t
deviations, 150
digital learning, 238
discussions, 153, 154, 216t
dissemination, 207–208
    conferences, 211–213
    creating plans, 208–209
    external, 211–217
    of findings, 66
    internal, 209–210
    projects, 228
    types of, 216–217
distribution of values, 150
documents

mission statements, 19–20
vision statements, 21

E

early adopters, 76b, 77f
early majority, 76b, 77f
economic evaluation, 175–177
education, 23, 26, 32, 48
    lessons learned, 65
    nurses, 9
effectiveness, 5
effective sizes, 152
effect size (ES), 142
efficacy, 5
efficiency, 5
electronic health records (EHRs), 201
elements
    application of PICO, 58f
    of strategic plans, 21f
Embase, 32, 254
Emergency Care Research Institute (ECRI), 167, 171
emergency department (ED), 174
EndNote, 116, 118
Enhancing the QUAlity and Transparency Of health Research (EQUATOR), 152, 170
environments
    building capacity, 29–33
    creating supportive, 13–15
    establishing organizational cultures, 19–29
    facilitating, 16
    interprofessional collaboration, 32–33
    planning communication, 35–37
    sustaining change, 33–35
EQUATOR Network, 215, 216
ERIC database, 238
ethnography, 140t

evaluation, 33, 61
    economic, 175–177
    of models, 16
    outcomes, 64–65
    of outcomes, 202–203
    program, 177
    searches, 115–118
    of statistical findings, 150–152
events, change, 26. *See also* change management
evidence, 59–62
    advanced search techniques, 114
    answerable questions, 101–102
    appraisal, 129 (*see also* research)
    central venous catheters (CVCs), 232–233
    classification systems, 121
    clinical practice guidelines (CPGs), 164–167
    collecting, 99
    creating EBP cultures, 241–242
    creating search strategies, 107–114
    databases as sources of, 100
    gamification in nursing education, 238–239
    Heat Charts, 197, 197f
    hierarchies, 121–123, 295–296
    Hierarchy of Evidence Guide, 123, 295–296
    individual, 60–61
    Individual Evidence Summary Tool, 124, 126, 266–267, 315–318
    integrative reviews, 168–170
    interpreting, 170–173
    JHNEBP Quality Rating scheme for Research Evidence, 233
    key information formats, 100–101
    learning through EBP projects, 224–225
    level of research in, 146–147
    literature reviews, 167–168
    multiple sources of, 163 (*see also* nonresearch)
    nonresearch (*see also* nonresearch)

Nonresearch Evidence Appraisal Tool,
    261–265, 307–314
overall body of, 61–62
PET (Practice Question, Evidence, and
    Translation), 51, 54–66
Physiotherapy Evidence Database
    (PEDro), 107
pressure injury prevention, 235–236
prevention of LVAD driveline infections,
    227
primary, 100
quality of, 60, 122, 147–160, 155–159
quality of life improvement, 230
quality of measurement, 147–150
recommendations, 61–62, 166t
Research Evidence Appraisal Tool, 160,
    254–260, 297–306
research summaries, 164–173
search examples, 102–103
searching, 29, 60, 99–100 (see also
    searching)
selecting resources, 104–106
selecting resources out of literature,
    106–107
strength of, 122
summaries, 124
synthesis, 124–126
Synthesis and Recommendations Tool,
    268–270, 319–323
tools, 254
type of, 142I–143t
evidence-based practice (EBP)
    access to information/library services, 31
    and accountability, 8–9
    answering questions, 172t–173t
    assimilation of, 22
    building capacity, 29–33
    clinical reasoning, 51–52
    creating cultures, 241–243
    critical thinking, 51–52
    decision trees, 92f
    defining problems, 83t–85t

definition of, 5
dissemination, 207–208 (see also
    dissemination)
environments, 13–15 (see also
    environments)
establishing organizational cultures,
    19–29
facilitating, 16
growth of, 7
healthcare clinician role in, 9
history of, 6–7
interprofessional collaboration, 32–33
interprofessional EBP teams, 74–80
knowledge and skills, 29–30
leadership, 17–19
mission statements, 19–20
need for, 15
need for projects, 90–95
outcomes and, 8
overcoming barriers, 24–25
overview of, 3–4
PET (Practice Question, Evidence, and
    Translation), 51, 54–66
planning communication, 35–37
processes, 33, 43–44
quality improvement (QI), 92–95
questions, 101 (see also questions)
requirements, 53–54
research, 92–95
roles of teams, 78–80
searching examples, 102–103
selecting models, 15–16
setting expectations, 34
sources of problems, 81t
structures of committees, 35t
success of, 22
sustaining change, 33–35
types of questions, 86–90
writing questions, 87–90
Evidence-Based Practice Centers (EPCs), 144
examples
    leveraging data, 125

meta-analysis, 143
meta-synthesis, 143
PICO (patient, intervention, comparison, outcomes), 102t, 103t
quasi-experimental studies, 136
searching, 102–103
summary vs. synthesis, 125
exclusion criteria, 117
executive summaries, 209
exemplars
  central venous catheters (CVCs), 231–234
  creating EBP cultures, 241–243
  gamification in nursing education, 237–240
  learning through EBP projects, 223–226
  pressure injury prevention, 234–237
  prevention of LVAD driveline infections, 226–228
  quality of life improvement, 229–231
expectations, setting, 34
experience, organizational, 173–181
  case reports, 178–179
  clinician experience, 179–180
  community standards, 179
  economic evaluation, 175–177
  expert opinions, 178
  patient/consumer experience, 180–181
  program evaluation, 177
  quality improvement (QI) reports, 173–175
experimental groups, 134
experimental research, 155–156
expert opinions, 178
external dissemination, 211–217
  conferences, 211–213
  peer-reviewed journal articles, 213–216
external factors, 53
external reviews, 167t
external searches, 60
external validity, 148

Facebook, 217
fast facts, 26
feasibility recommendations, 196–198
feedback, 7, 20, 23, 198
filters, databases, 109
findings
  disseminating, 66
  evaluating statistical, 150–152
  interventions, 103
  lessons learned, 65
  research, 101 (*see also* research)
  synthesizing, 61
fit recommendations, 196–198
Food and Drug Administration, 53
foreground questions, 86–90
formal education, 49
formats, information, 100–101
free online resources, 111t–112t
free resources, 107–114
The Future of Nursing: Leading Change, Advancing Health (2011), 15

gamification, 237–240
Generation Y, 15
Generation Z, 15
generic descriptive, 141t
goals, 21
  Institute of Medicine (IOM), 43
  SMART, 194, 194t, 201
Google Scholar, 113–114, 235
Grading of Recommendations, Assessment, Development and Evaluations (GRADE), 164
graphics, 213

grounded theory, 140t
group collaboration, 50
guidelines, 6, 7, 29
    clinical practice guidelines (CPGs), 164–167
    development groups, 164
    Johns Hopkins Evidence-Based Practice Model and Guidelines, 122f
    National Guideline Clearinghouse, 171
    practices, 14
    Systematic Reviews and Meta-Analyses (PRISMA), 117
    updating, 167t

Health and Psychosocial Instruments (HaPI), 107
Health Business Full Text, 101
healthcare
    accountability in, 8–9
    clinician role in evidence-based practice (EBP), 9
    consumers and, 180–181
    environments, 13 (see also environments)
    evidence-based practice (EBP) in, 6 (see also evidence-based practice [EBP])
    healthcare systems, 3
    practices, 14
    team members, 25
Healthcare Cost and Utilization Project (HCUP), 100
healthcare professionals (HCPs). See also nurses
    clinical reasoning, 51–52
    components (of JHEBP), 44
    core competencies, 47f
    critical thinking, 51–52
    definition of inquiry, 45
    EVB processes, 43–44
    learning, 48–49
    practice, 45–48
    standards, 46
Health Consumer Assessment of Healthcare Providers and Systems (HCAHPS), 52
health inequity, 171
Health Professions Education: A Bridge to Quality (2003), 14, 46
Health Resources and Services Administration (HRSA), 32, 113
Heat Charts, 197, 197f
hierarchies
    evidence, 121–123, 295–296
    Johns Hopkins Evidence-Based Practice Model and Guidelines, 122f
Hierarchy of Evidence Guide, 123, 295–296
hospitals, communication strategies, 209

images, 213
impact
    factors, 214
    of projects, 78
implementation, 190, 242. See also translation
    action plans, 200–201, 202
    plans, 24
    science, 191b
    teams, 31
improvement, models for, 195f
incentives, lack of, 25
InCites Journal Citation Reports, 214
inclusion criteria, 117
independent variables, 134
indexers, 105
individual evidence, 60–61
Individual Evidence Summary Tool, 60, 266–267, 315–318

informal leaders
　characteristics of, 78*t*
　developing, 22–23 (*see also* leadership)
informal learning sources, 31
information
　formats, 100–101
　literacy, 99
　selecting resources, 104–106
infrastructure, lack of organizational, 25
innovation, 23
innovators, 76*b*
inquiry
　components (of JHEBP), 45
　definition of, 45
　selecting forms of, 95*f*
　as starting point for JHEBP Model, 51
　three forms of, 93*t*
inquiry-learning process, 49, 50
Institute of Medicine (IOM), 3, 14, 32
　clinical practice guidelines (CPGs), 164–167
　Clinical Practice Guidelines We Can Trust (2011), 170
　Consensus Study, 74
　Crossing the Quality Chasm (2001), 14
　The Future of Nursing: Leading Change, Advancing Health (2011), 15
　goals, 43
　Health Professions Education: A Bridge to Quality (2003), 14, 46
　Roundtable on Evidence-Based Medicine (2009), 15
　Standards for Trustworthy Guidelines, 167
Institutional Review Board (IRB), 123
integrative reviews, 168–170
internal consistency, 151*t*
internal dissemination, 209–210
internal factors, 53
internal searches, 60
internal validity, 147

International Academy of Nursing Editors (INANE), 214
interpreting evidence, 170–173
interpretive descriptive, 141*t*
interprofessional collaboration, 32–33
interprofessional EBP teams, 74–80
Interprofessional Education Collaborative (IPEC), 32
interprofessional leaders, recommendations for, 160
interprofessional teams, recruiting, 55
interrater reliability, 151*t*
intervention, 57, 88, 89, 90, 103. See also PICO
introductions, 153, 216*t*
investigator bias, 149*t*

J

JBI, 6, 101, 106, 145*t*, 254
JHNEBP Nonresearch Evidence Appraisal Tool, 176
JHNEBP Quality Rating scheme for Research Evidence, 233
Joanna Briggs Institute. *See* JBI
job descriptions, 34
Johns Hopkins Evidence-Based Practice Model (JHEBP), 5, 9, 29, 44*f*, 122*f*. *See also* evidence-based practice (EBP)
　components, 44–49
　description of, 49–54
　factors influencing, 53–54
　implementation teams, 31
　Model for Nurses and HCPs, 43–44 (*see also* healthcare professionals (HCPs); nurses)
　PET (Practice Question, Evidence, and Translation), 51, 54–66, 55*f* (*see also* Practice Question, Evidence, and Translation [PET])

Johns Hopkins Evidence-Based Practice (JHNEBP) Question Development Tool, 74
The Johns Hopkins Hospital (JHH), 20, 223, 247
Johns Hopkins Welch Library, 232
Johnson's Behavioral System Model, 135
Joint Commission, 47, 53
Josiah Macy Jr. Foundation, 32
Josie King Foundation, 181
Journal/Author Name Estimator, 214
journals, 4
    peer-reviewed journal articles, 213–216
    predatory, 215
    Worldviews on Evidence-Based Nursing, 7

key information formats, 100–101
keywords, 108
    searching, 224, 227
    selecting, 109
knowledge. *See also* education
    dissemination (*see* dissemination)
    evidence-based practice (EBP), 29–30
    internalizing complex, 50
knowledge-to-action models, 192*t*

laggards, 76*b*, 77*f*
late majority, 76*b*, 77*f*
laws, 53
leadership
    characteristics of informal leaders, 78*t*
    commitments, 19
    communication strategies, 209
    core practices of, 79–80
    cultures and, 19 (*see also* cultures)
    developing informal leaders, 22–23
    developing mentors, 22–23
    dissemination, 208
    evidence-based practice (EBP), 17–19
    lack of supportive, 24
    opinion leaders, 23, 200
    recommendations for healthcare leaders, 182–183
    recommendations for interprofessional leaders, 160
    responsibilities of, 24, 56
    selecting EBP models, 16
    support and visibility of, 18
    transition strategies, 27–29
learning. *See also* education
    components (of JHEBP), 48–49
    cultures, 48
    definition of, 48
    lessons learned, 65
legislation, 53
lessons learned, 65
let it happen approach, 17, 26
libraries
    access to services, 31
    catalogs, 100
    Cochrane Library, 100, 101, 106
    National Library of Medicine (NM), 104, 112, 113
lifelong learning, 13
literacy, information, 99
literature
    databases, 32, 101
    reviews, 167–168
    searching, 254 (*see also* databases)
    selecting resources outside of, 106–107
    shortcomings of available, 168
    translation, 101
longitudinal studies, 136
loss, assessing, 27

M

Magnet Certification, 48
Magnet Recognition Program, 53
make it happen approach, 18
management
  commitments, 19
  communication strategies, 209
  cultures and, 19 (*see also* cultures)
  developing mentors, 22–23
  dissemination, 208
  evidence-based practice (EBP), 17–19
  opinion leaders, 23, 200
  recommendations for healthcare leaders, 182–183
  recommendations for interprofessional leaders, 160
  responsibilities of, 24
  risks, 63
  selecting EBP models, 16
  styles, 17
  support and visibility of, 18
  transitions, 26–27
  transition strategies, 27–29
Managing Transitions: Making the Most of Change (Bridges and Bridges), 199
manipulation, 134, 135. *See also* intervention
manuscripts
  components of submissions, 216*t*
  pathway to publication, 214*f*
  submission, 213
McMaster University Medical School (Canada), 6
McMillan, Mary, 6
mean, 150
meaning, team roles and, 78
measurement
  of central tendency, 150
  quality of, 147–150
  statistical significance, 152
  types of outcome measures, 202*t*–203*t*
medians, 150
medical intensive care unit (MICU), 174
Medical Subject Headings (MeSH), 105, 168, 235
MEDLINE, 4, 104–105, 232, 235
meetings, scheduling, 56, 80
Melnyk's Scale, 243
Mendeley, 116
mentors
  developing, 22–23
  roles of, 22–23
messages. *See also* communication
  developing, 36
  dissemination, 208 (*see also* dissemination)
meta-analysis, systematic reviews with, 142–143, 158–159
meta-synthesis, systematic reviews with, 143, 159
methods, 153–154, 209, 216*t*
metrics, 89
millennials, 15
mission statements, 19–20, 20*b*
mixed-methods
  research, 131
  studies, 145–146
models
  Agency for Healthcare Research and Quality (AHRQ), 192*t*
  development of, 6
  evidence-based practice, 9 (*see also* evidence-based practice [EBP])
  for improvement, 195*f*
  Johnson's Behavioral System Model, 135
  knowledge-to-action, 192*t*
  PARIHS, 192*t*
  Plan-Do-Study-Act (PDSA), 174, 175, 191, 193–195
  QUERI implementation roadmap, 193*t*

RE-AIM, 193t
selecting, 15–16
staffing, 176
translation, 190–195
modes, 150
monitoring, 177. *See also* evaluation
My NCBI, 116

narrative inquiry, 140t
narrative reviews, 142
National Academies of Sciences, Engineering, and Medicine, 14
National Academy of Medicine (NAM), 3, 14
National Center for Advancing Translational Sciences, 9
National Guideline Clearinghouse (NGC), 167, 171
National Health Service (Great Britain), 6
National Institutes of Health (NIH), 9, 113
National League for Nursing (NLN), 45, 104
National Library of Medicine (NLM), 104, 112, 113
National Magnet Conference (ANCC [2019]), 211
natural experiments, 138, 139t
need for EBP projects, 90–95
negative correlations, 138
Nightingale, Florence, 6
non-experimental research, 133t, 136, 157–158
nonresearch, 163
  best practices companies, 182
  case reports, 178–179
  clinical practice guidelines (CPGs), 164–167

clinician experience, 179–180
community standards, 179
economic evaluation, 175–177
expert opinions, 178
integrative reviews, 168–170
interpreting evidence, 170–173
literature reviews, 167–168
organizational experience, 173–181
patient/consumer experience, 180–181
program evaluation, 177
quality improvement (QI) reports, 173–175
recommendations for healthcare leaders, 182–183
research summaries, 164–173
Nonresearch Evidence Appraisal Tool, 60, 179, 261–265, 307–314
NOT operator, 108, 109, 110t
nurse managers (NMs), 18
Nurse Practice Act, 53
nurses
  components (of JHEBP), 44–49
  education, 9
  EVB processes, 43–44
nursing
  protocols, 6, 7
  selecting resources out of literature, 106–107
  state boards of, 53
  structures of committees, 35t
  three forms of inquiry, 93t

objectives, 21, 29, 30t
one-day workshops, 29, 30t
operators, Boolean, 108, 109, 110t, 168
opinion leaders, 23, 200
organizational cultures, 53, 199

organizational experience, 173–181
  case reports, 178–179
  clinician experience, 179–180
  community standards, 179
  economic evaluation, 175–177
  expert opinions, 178
  patient/consumer experience, 180–181
  program evaluation, 177
  quality improvement (QI) reports, 173–175
OR operator, 108, 109, 110*t*
outcomes
  definition of, 89*t*
  evaluating, 64–65, 202–203
  and evidence-based practice (EBP), 8
  learning through EBP projects, 225–226
  PICO, 57, 88, 89, 90 (*see also* PICO)
  types of outcome measures, 202*t*–203*t*
Outcomes Measurement Plan, 64

P

Papers, 116
PARIHS model, 192*t*
Patient-Centered Outcomes Research Institute (PCORI), 181
patients
  definition of care, 45
  experience, 180–181
  outcomes, 8 (*see also* outcomes)
  PICO, 57 (*see also* PICO)
  preferences, 5, 7
pay-for-performance initiatives, 14
Pearson, Alan, 6
Pediatric Intensive Care Unit (PICU) adopter curves, 77*f*
peer-reviewed journal articles, 213–216
performance, feedback, 23
phenomenology, 140*t*

philosophies, 20
Physiotherapy Evidence Database (PEDro), 107
PICO (patient, intervention, comparison, outcomes), 57, 58*t*, 88, 89, 90, 232
  examples, 102*t*, 103*t*
  foreground questions, 90*t*
pictures, 213
Plan-Do-Study-Act (PDSA), 64, 65, 94, 174, 175, 191, 193–195, 227, 228
planning
  Action Planning Tool, 271–275
  action plans, 63–64
  communication, 35–37
  developing strategic plans, 21
  dissemination, 207–208 (*see also* dissemination)
  review cycle of policies, 247
  Translation and Action Planning Tool, 325–332
Plus, 32
policies, 7, 247
population (PICO), 57, 88, 89, 90. *See also* PICO
position statements, 164–167
positive correlations, 138
poster presentations, 211, 212
PowerPoint, 212. *See also* poster presentations
practice
  change, 47, 90
  clarifying/describing problems, 80–85
  clinical practice guidelines (CPGs), 164–167
  components (of JHEBP), 45–48
  dissemination (*see* dissemination)
  guidelines, 14
  healthcare, 14
  PET (Practice Question, Evidence, and Translation), 51, 54–66
  setting-specific recommendations, 196

strengthening, 18
translating evidence into, 9
Practice Question, Evidence, and Translation (PET), 51, 54–66. *See also* evidence; practice question phase (PET); translation
 exemplars (*see* exemplars)
 Process Guide, 248–249, 279–282
 tools (*see* tools)
practice question phase (PET), 73–74
 central venous catheters (CVCs), 231–232
 clarifying/describing practice problems, 80–85
 creating EBP cultures, 241
 developing/refining EBP questions, 86
 gamification in nursing education, 237–238
 identifying stakeholders, 95–96
 interprofessional EBP teams, 74–80
 learning through EBP projects, 223–224
 need for EBP projects, 90–95
 pressure injury prevention, 234–235
 prevention of LVAD driveline infections, 226–227
 quality of life improvement, 229
 review cycle of policies, 247
 selecting background/foreground questions, 86–90
 steps in, 74*b*
practice setting-specific recommendations, 62–63
predatory journals, 215
presentations
 podium, 212–213
 poster, 211, 212
preventive services, 14
primary evidence, 100
PRISMA diagrams, 227
problems
 clarifying/describing practice, 80–85
 defining, 83*t*–85*t*
 PICO, 57, 88, 89, 90 (*see also* PICO)
 sources of, 81*t*

statements, 82
problem-solving, 5. *See also* evidence-based practice (EBP)
processes
 definition of, 89*t*
 dissemination (*see* dissemination)
 evidence-based practice (EBP), 43–44
 inquiry-learning, 49, 50
 peer-reviewed journal articles, 213
 PET (Practice Question, Evidence, and Translation), 51
 reviewing, 65
 writing (*see* writing)
Process Guide (PET), 248–249, 279–282
program evaluation, 177
PROGRESS-Plus, 171
projects
 decision trees, 92*f*
 dissemination, 207–208, 228 (*see also* dissemination)
 impact of, 78
 leadership responsibilities, 56
 need for EBP, 58–59, 90–95
 review cycle of policies, 247
prospective studies, 136
protocols, nursing, 6, 7
psychological safety, 78
PsycINFO, 32, 106–107
Publication Guide, 276, 334–336
publication standards, 213
PubMed, 32, 100, 101, 104–105, 108, 224, 235, 238, 254
 clinical queries, 105
 filters, 109
 storing searches, 116
purposes of dissemination, 207, 208
p-values, 152

Q

qualitative research, 130, 140–141, 157–158
qualitative systematic reviews, 169*t*
quality
 of evidence, 60, 122, 147–160, 155–159
 of measurement, 147–150
 Plan-Do-Study-Act (PDSA), 64, 65
 of reporting, 152–154
Quality Assurance Performance Improvement (QAPI), 228
quality improvement (QI), 92–95, 123, 193, 224, 227
 reports, 173–175
quantitative research, 130
quasi-experimental research, 132*t*, 135–136, 156–157
queries, clinical queries (PubMed), 105
QUERI implementation roadmap, 193*t*
Question Development Tool, 58, 101, 102, 250–251, 283–288
questions
 answerable, 101–102
 attributes to answer EBP, 172*t*–173*t*
 clinical, 82
 developing and refining, 57–58
 developing/refining EBP, 86
 Johns Hopkins Evidence-Based Practice (JHNEBP) Question Development Tool, 74
 PET (Practice Question, Evidence, and Translation), 51, 54–66
 practice, 55–59
 questioning, 36
 reflective, 50
 selecting background/foreground, 86–90
 writing EBP, 87–90

R

random control trials (RCT), 224
randomization, 134
ranges of values, 152
rapid cycle quality improvement (QI), 193
rapid reviews, 169*t*
ratings
 JHNEBP Quality Rating scheme for Research Evidence, 233
 level of research evidence, 146*t*–147*t*
 quality of evidence, 155*t*
RE-AIM model, 193*t*
recognition, lack of, 25
recommendations, 166*t*
 acceptability, 196
 clinical practice guidelines (CPGs), 164–167
 evidence, 61–62
 feasibility, 196–198
 fit, 196–198
 for healthcare leaders, 182–183
 for interprofessional leaders, 160
 practice setting-specific, 62–63, 196
 Synthesis and Recommendations Tool, 268–270, 319–323
records, 4
recruiting interprofessional teams, 55
reflective questions, 50
RefWorks, 116
regulations, 53
reliability of research, 149–150
reporting
 quality of, 152–154
 Standards for Quality Improvement Reporting Excellence (SQUIRE), 174
reports
 case, 178–179
 Crossing the Quality Chasm14 (2001), 14

The Future of Nursing: Leading Change, Advancing Health (2011), 15
Health Professions Education: A Bridge to Quality (2003), 14, 46
    quality improvement (QI), 173–175
    results to stakeholders, 65
Roundtable on Evidence-Based Medicine (2009), 15
requirements (EBP), 53–54
research, 9, 24, 33, 92–95
    clinical practice guidelines (CPGs), 164–167
    correlational studies, 138–139
    descriptive studies, 137–138
    designs, 131–141
    differentiating levels, 123
    evidence-based practice (EBP), 92–95
    experimental, 155–156
    information formats, 100–101
    information literacy and, 99
    integrative reviews, 168–170
    interpreting evidence, 170–173
    level of evidence in, 146–147
    literature reviews, 167–168
    mixed-methods, 131
    non-experimental, 133*t*, 136, 157–158
    nonresearch, 163 (*see also* nonresearch)
    qualitative, 130, 140–141, 157–158
    quality of evidence, 147–160
    quality of measurement, 147–150
    quantitative, 130
    quasi-experimental, 132*t*, 135–136, 156–157
    reliability of, 149–150
    single studies, 132–141
    summaries, 141–146, 164–173
    true experimental, 132*t*, 133–135
    types of, 130
    univariate, 133*t*
    univariate research, 139–140
    validity of, 147–149

Research Evidence Appraisal Tool, 60, 160, 176, 254–260, 297–306
Research Portfolio Online Reporting Tool (RePORTER), 113
resistance to change, 26
resources
    action plan implementation, 200–201, 202
    for action plans, 64
    free, 107–114 (*see also* free resources)
    outside of nursing literature, 106–107
    selecting, 104–106
    systematic reviews, 144–145
Respiratory Care Scope of Practice (2018), 46
responsibilities of leadership, 24, 56
results, 153, 154, 216*t*
    storing search, 115–118
retrospective studies, 136
reviewing
    critical reviews, 169*t*
    integrative reviews, 168–170
    literature reviews, 167–168
    narrative reviews, 142
    peer-reviewed journal articles, 213–216
    policies, 247
    processes, 65
    qualitative systematic reviews, 169*t*
    rapid reviews, 169*t*
    research summaries, 141–146
    scoping reviews, 169*t*
    searches, 116–117
    state-of-the-art reviews, 170*t*
    systematic reviews, 158, 166*t*
    systematized reviews, 170*t*
revisions, searching, 109, 115–118
rewards, lack of, 25
risks, 5
    Heat Charts, 197, 197*f*
    management, 63

Robert Wood Johnson Foundation, 32
  best practices study (2015), 75
roles
  of healthcare clinicians, 9
  of mentors, 22–23
  of teams, 78–80
Roundtable on Evidence-Based Medicine (2009), 15

S

safety, Heat Charts, 197, 197f
sample sizes, 152
scenario-based, 238
scheduling meetings, 56, 80
science, implementation, 191b
scientific research, 130. *See also* research
scoping reviews, 169t
screening, 117, 118
searching
  advanced search techniques, 114
  articles, 235
  biases, 100, 103
  Boolean operators, 108, 109, 110t, 168
  classification systems, 121
  creating search strategies, 107–114
  evaluating, 115–118
  evidence, 29, 99–100
  for evidence, 60
  examples, 102–103
  exclusion criteria, 117
  hierarchies, 121–123
  inclusion criteria, 117
  for interventions, 103
  keywords, 108, 224, 227
  literature, 254 (*see also* databases)
  revisions, 109
  spelling variations, 109
selection bias, 149t
Sigma Repository, 112

single study research, 132–141
skills
  clinical reasoning, 51–52
  critical thinking, 51–52, 61
  evidence-based practice (EBP), 29–30
  information literacy, 99 (*see also* searching)
slides, 213. *See also* presentations
SMART goals, 194, 194t, 201
social media, 217
Solomon 4 group, 133, 134
spelling variations, 109
staffing models, 176
Stakeholder Analysis and Communication Tool, 252–253, 289–293
stakeholders, 201
  dissemination, 208
  identifying, 59, 95–96
  reporting results to, 65
standard deviations, 150
standards, 6
  clinical practice guidelines (CPGs), 166t–167t
  community, 179
  EQUATOR Network, 215, 216
  healthcare professionals (HCPs), 46
  publication, 213
  Respiratory Care Scope of Practice (2018), 46
  standardization of practices, 228
Standards for Quality Improvement Reporting Excellence (SQUIRE), 174
Standards of Practice for Clinical Pharmacists (2014), 46
state boards of nursing, 53
statements
  consensus statements (CSs), 165
  mission, 19–20
  position, 164–167
  problem, 82
  vision, 21

state-of-the-art reviews, 170t
statistical findings, evaluating, 150–152
statistical significance, 152
storage, search results, 115–118
strategies, 4. *See also* evidence-based practice (EBP)
   communication, 209–210
   creating search, 107–114
   defining EBP problems, 83t–85t
   developing strategic plans, 21
   dissemination, 208 (*see also* dissemination)
   Grading of Recommendations, Assessment, Development and Evaluations (GRADE) strategy, 164
   transitions, 27–29
strength of evidence, 122
structures
   definition of, 89t
   of teams, 78
submission
   manuscripts, 213
   pathway to publication, 214f
Substance Abuse and Mental Health Services Administration (SAMHSA), 113
success of evidence-based practice (EBP), 22
summaries
   creating EBP cultures, 243
   evidence, 124
   executive, 209
   gamification in nursing education, 240
   Individual Evidence Summary Tool, 266–267, 315–318
   interpreting evidence, 170–173
   pressure injury prevention, 237
   prevention of LVAD driveline infections, 228
   quality of life improvement, 231
   research, 141–146, 164–173
support
   action plan implementation, 200–201, 202
   for action plans, 64
sustainability
   of communication, 36
   sustaining change, 33–35
synthesis, 52, 61
   evidence, 124–126
   systematic reviews with meta-synthesis, 143, 159
Synthesis and Recommendations Tool, 268–270, 319–323
systematic reviews, 158, 166t
   with meta-analysis, 142–143, 158–159
   with meta-synthesis, 143, 159
   mixed-method studies, 145–146
   research summaries, 141–146
   sources of, 144–145
Systematic Reviews and Meta-Analyses (PRISMA) guidelines, 117
systematized reviews, 170t

T

teams
   change, 28
   clarity of, 78
   identifying collaboration, 75
   implementation, 31
   interprofessional EBP, 74–80
   meaning, 78
   members, 25
   recruiting interprofessional, 55
   role of, 78–80
   scheduling meetings, 56
   structure of, 78
templates
   for presentations, 212
   text, 216
test-retest reliability, 151t
text
   for presentations, 213

templates, 216
writing (*see* writing)
timing of dissemination, 208
titles, 153
    searching, 117
    title pages, 216*t*
tools, 247
    Action Planning Tool, 271–275
    Appraisal of Guidelines for Research and Evaluation (AGREE) II, 233
    Appraisal of Guidelines Research and Evaluation (AGREE) Collaboration, 165, 166
    communicating change, 200*t*
    evidence, 254
    Hierarchy of Evidence Guide, 123, 295–296
    Individual Evidence Summary Tool, 60, 124, 126, 266–267, 315–318
    JHNEBP Nonresearch Evidence Appraisal Tool, 176
    Johns Hopkins Evidence-Based Practice (JHNEBP) Question Development Tool, 74
    Nonresearch Evidence Appraisal Tool, 60, 179, 261–265, 307–314
    Process Guide (PET), 248–249, 279–282
    Publication Guide, 276, 334–336
    Question Development Tool, 58, 101, 102, 250–251, 283–288
    Research Evidence Appraisal Tool, 60, 160, 176, 254–260, 297–306
    Stakeholder Analysis and Communication Tool, 252–253, 289–293
    Synthesis and Recommendations Tool, 268–270, 319–323
    translation, 271
    Translation and Action Planning Tool, 63, 64, 325–332
topics, one-day workshops, 29, 30*t*
transformational learning, 48

transitions, 17, 20
    definition of, 26*t*
    managing, 26–27
    strategies, 27–29
translation, 62, 189–190
    action plan implementation, 200–201, 202
    Action Planning Tool, 271–275
    action plans, 63–64, 198–200
    central venous catheters (CVCs), 233–234
    communicating change, 200*t*
    components of translation phase, 196–203
    creating EBP cultures, 242–243
    disseminating findings, 66
    evaluating outcomes, 64–65
    gamification in nursing education, 240
    implementing action plans, 64
    learning through EBP projects, 225
    literature, 101
    models, 190–195
    PET (Practice Question, Evidence, and Translation), 51, 54–66
    Plan-Do-Study-Act (PDSA), 193–195
    practice setting-specific recommendations, 62–63
    pressure injury prevention, 236
    prevention of LVAD driveline infections, 227–228
    Publication Guide, 276, 334–336
    quality of life improvement, 230–231
    reporting results to stakeholders, 65
    resources/support for action plans, 64
    SMART goals, 194, 194*t*
    tools, 271
Translation and Action Planning Tool, 63, 64, 325–332
transparency, 28, 166*t*
    lack of (journals), 215
TRIP Medical Database, 112
troubleshooting, 193

true experimental research, 132t, 133–135
TRUST (Transparency and Rigor Using Standards of Trustworthiness), 167
Twitter, 217
types
　of dissemination, 216–217
　of literature review, 169t–170t
　of outcome measures, 202t–203t
　of research, 130–131

univariate research, 133t, 139–140
US Department of Veterans Affairs (VA), 113
US Preventive Services Task Force (USPSTF), 14, 112

validity (of research), 147–149
values
　distribution of, 150
　ranges of, 152
variables, 134
variations, 142
Virginia Henderson Global Nursing e-Repository. *See* Sigma Repository
vision statements, 21
vocabularies
　CINAHL, 104
　controlled, 108
　keywords, 108
　Medical Subject Headings (MeSH), 105

Web of Science, 32
Work Breakdown Structure (WBS), 332
workshops, 29, 30t
World Health Organization (WHO), 121, 165
Worldviews on Evidence-Based Nursing, 7
writing
　EBP questions, 87–90
　hints, 217b
　manuscripts (*see* manuscripts)
　peer-reviewed journal articles, 213

YouTube, 217

zero correlations, 138
Zotero, 116